Caregiving Ties That Bind

Today's Caregiver Magazine
Celebrity Interviews

Caregiving Ties That Bind

Today's Caregiver™ Magazine
Celebrity Interviews

GARY BARG
Editor-in-Chief, Today's Caregiver magazine

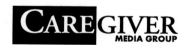

First paperback edition 2013

Caregiver.com™
3350 Griffin Road
Ft. Lauderdale, FL. 33312-5519
www.caregiver.com

ISBN 978-0-9834066-1-7

Designed by Adnan Razack & Melody Capielo
Cover Design by Doralee Mendez

First Edition
10 9 8 7 6 5

CONTENTS

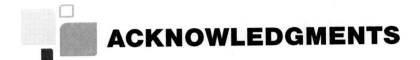

ACKNOWLEDGMENTS

Thanks to all of the celebrity caregivers you will meet within these pages for letting us peek behind the curtain to share their personal stories with us. Thanks to my partners Nancy Schonwalter and Steven Barg and our exquisite staff for making everything we do for family caregivers possible. Thanks to Christian T. Andaya and Morris Barg for making everything else possible. Thanks to Robert M. Barg and Joseph Weiss for the love that they engendered in their entire extended family. Thanks to Monica M. Barg for showing me the heart of caregiving so many years ago and, most especially, thanks to the thousands of family caregivers I have learned so much from over these past seventeen years, as well as those caregivers I have yet to meet and the lessons that they will also share with me.

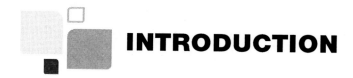

INTRODUCTION

My brother, Steven, is a terrific cook. The dishes he prepares range as far and wide as the places he lived in when he worked in the shopping mall industry before he became publisher of *Today's Caregiver* magazine. His job was to rehabilitate old and decrepit shopping malls for the owners who, upon renewal, usually sold the facilities. This position meant that he would live in the cities where these malls were located for a few years at a time. Luckily, they were usually great food meccas of the south, including Georgia, North Carolina and even New Orleans, Louisiana. The skills that he has as a chef must be in part genetic; our mom is and both grandmothers were excellent chefs. I must have missed out on this genetic trait since I have been known to actually burn water. My culinary abilities are more in the field of being a highly appreciative diner. And I can clean a mean kitchen. This came in handy in the years that Steven and I lived together after college. He ascribes to the notion that a kitchen should groan under the efforts that went into any meal worthy of comment. Our mom still marvels at how he was able to get tomato sauce on the kitchen ceiling after one particularly inspired Italian dinner.

It is no great surprise when I find him engaged in recipe swapping with the folks we meet on the road while hosting our Fearless Caregiver Conferences. I usually walk away as he and his fellow connoisseurs talk about oven temperatures, seasonings and baking times. One such conversation does stand out, however. It was in a ready room at the Los Angeles Convention Center before the start of that day's Fearless Caregiver Conference. To date, our company has produced over a hundred of these highly interactive events around the nation.

The conversation I walked in on that day was with Grammy award winning legend Della Reese. Della has been the keynote speaker at three Fearless Caregiver Conferences over the years and graced the cover of *Today's Caregiver* magazine when she gave an interview in which she spoke frankly about her life with diabetes and as a family caregiver. That morning, Steven and Della were talking about her recipe for navy bean pie and her story was as funny as the recipe was mouthwatering. She later shared personal caregiving stories with a room filled with 400 family caregivers. Although the topic of green bean pie did not arise, she fielded many questions about her caregiving and taking care of herself as a person living with diabetes with grace and honesty. The same situation has played out at every Fearless Caregiver Conference in which we had a celebrity caregiver as a keynote speaker. In Cleveland and Phoenix, caregivers asked Debbie Reynolds about caring for her mom, not the making of *Singing in the Rain* or the *Tammy* movies. My concept is that when you bring 400 family caregivers and a celebrity who is or has been a family caregiver together, what you actually have is a room filled with 401 family caregivers. Caring for and about our loved ones are the ties that bind us all together.

It was actually my other sibling that I have to thank for the opportunity to interview over 100 celebrity caregivers and caregiving advocates—my sister, Linda. In 1995, when the first copies of *Today's Caregiver* rolled off the presses, she started lobbying for us to include celebrity cover interviews in each issue. Frankly, I thought it was a terrible idea. I was convinced that family caregivers would react negatively to hearing the stories about the rich and famous caring for their loved ones. In fact, nothing could be further from the truth. Finally, in the third issue of the magazine, we ran our first celebrity cover interview and the response was tremendous—a fact she never lets me forget.

My own journey as a family caregiver started many years ago as I helped my mom care for my dad who retired in 1990 at the age of 59 and within three months, was diagnosed with bone marrow cancer. Mom went from business partner, traveling partner, best friend and spouse to being a full-time caregiver as his condition worsened. He passed away a year and a half later and immediately afterwards, Mom become caregiver for her parents who were with, respectively, cancer, Alzheimer's, diabetes, and strokes. At the time, I was living in a different state, and spoke with her on the phone every week. She never asked me to return home, but I knew by the distress in her voice during one of our conversations that things were not as rosy as she had been presenting. During the waning days of summer in 1994, I had the opportunity to go home for two weeks. I planned to be there long enough to help Mom make some decisions concerning my grandparents, look over some paperwork, offer support, and be back on my way to Atlanta, where I was living and working as a video producer, getting ready to produce work for the upcoming 1996 Olympics. Yet, before I unpacked my suitcase on the first day of my visit home, things were already in full swing. We received a call from the facility where my grandfather was living. He had been in an assisted living facility for the past two years and recently, his behavior had changed to the point where more oversight was necessary and the facility was insistent that we move him immediately. My grandmother had taken a fall, which combined with her intense depression and strokes, made the multiple doctor visits necessary for her care a physical challenge for Mom. At the end of my two week visit, as Mom and I sat on the couch in her house exhausted from the constant challenges presented by caring for our family members, I turned to her and said, "You know, I'm glad that I was able to visit during these particular two weeks due to all that went on." She looked at me blankly and asked, "What are you talking about?" It dawned on me that while I thought these two weeks represented an unusually intense and painful roller-coaster ride of healthcare, financial and mental challenges, to Mom, it was just another few weeks in her life as a caregiver.

I returned to Atlanta long enough to gather my belongings and move back home for the duration. I had become what I like to call a caregiver's caregiver. I was going to do whatever was necessary to support Mom as she helped to make our relatives' lives as comfortable and as safe as possible. A few months later, after visiting my grandmother during one of her many hospital stays, I had lunch in a restaurant on Miami Beach. In front of me on the restaurant table was spread the mountains of paperwork I had to sort through as a caregiver. These included flyers from the Alzheimer's Association, brochures from a variety of Assisted Living Facilities and a huge pile of insurance papers. It occurred to me that there must be a better way to organize this information for caregivers and that they deserved all the help that could be found. Although my background was in video and film, it seemed that a magazine was a better media to create in order to more quickly distribute to caregivers in need. But first, I would have to do some research. It was utterly impossible that there wouldn't already be such a publication out there. Bankers had magazines, floor manufacturers had magazines; there certainly must have already been a magazine available for family caregivers. Over the next few weeks, I looked in every library and bookstore in the area (this was before Internet search engines) and could find nothing. A year later, I watched as the first issue of *Today's Caregiver* magazine rolled off the presses.

The next 17 years quickly flew by. I have been blessed to meet many dedicated and loving family caregivers over these years, either online at caregiver.com or at our Fearless Caregiver Conferences. And many of these loving caregivers and care advocates are represented in the interviews in the pages of this book.

It has been and remains an honor to be able to share these stories with our magazine readers and visitors to caregiver.com. I also believe that it is a refreshing change for our cover celebrities from the traditional interview tours in which they talk about their latest movie or album to a vast array of media outlets. I feel that these interviews about their own family caregiving allow them to step out from behind the persona and share personal stories about themselves and their loved ones. My sister got it exactly right.

Hearing Dixie Cartier talk about the anguish of caring for her beloved father or Dana Reeve talk about the techniques that she had to create on the fly to deal with insurance company challenges or listening to Barbara Eden share the pain she still feels regarding her son's drug addiction and eventual suicide make us all closer as family caregivers. It shows us that family caregiving is one experience that challenges us all and no amount of money or fame erases the depth of pain that every single loving caregiver feels, regardless if the statue on the mantel is an Oscar or a bowling league trophy. In these pages, we have gathered some of the most interesting and significant celebrity cover interviews from *Today's Caregiver* magazine over the past 17 years, as well as some previously unshared stories about our fellow caregivers with the famous faces.

As caregivers, there is much to be learned from any conversation with another family caregiver, whether it is in a pharmacy waiting line with a neighbor or hearing the personal stories from these caregivers who also entertain, educate and motivate us through our CD players, on the silver screen or even through our television sets. So many times, behind the greasepaint and away from the bright lights, they also have loved ones for whom they care and face many of the emotional challenges that we all face on a daily basis. I have enjoyed sharing these conversations and look forward to many more. I believe that the open, honest and heart-felt stories told by the celebrities in this book are, indeed, the ties that bind us all together as family caregivers.

Caregiver
ADVOCATES

Life is much too short to be angry. Life is much too short to not love and be loved. There are some people who say, "I'll never be loved," but I think if we give the love first, it will come back to us.

— Lauren Chapin

GARY'S NOTE: DELLA REESE

Della Reese was the keynote speaker at a Philadelphia Fearless Caregiver Conference which was held at the Union League Center in downtown Philadelphia.

Late in the day, a caregiver who had been sitting silently for most of the day raised her hand to speak. She told us that her mother was in the hospital getting prepped for surgery, but she knew being with us was too important for her to miss. She said that she was the sole informal caregiver for six of her neighbors and she had two heart attacks in the past two years. Della and the audience members gave her advice and support until a caregiver from across the room said, "I live in your neighborhood and from now on, you're not alone." Tears flowed from every eye in the room. At the next year's event, these caregivers were sitting beside each other and told the spellbound room of their accomplishments in their neighborhood over the past year.

There are two more things about that event with Della Reese that I would like to share with you. The first was that three weeks after the event, I received an email out of the blue from a family caregiver who was bemoaning the fact that no one in her community would ever know what she went through as a caregiver and was convinced she was absolutely alone in her fears and concerns. The upshot of that story is that she lives not three miles from the Union League. The second was our amusement with the caregiver who would constantly refer to Della Reese as Ella (as in Fitzgerald). Finally, Della was moved to say, chuckling and in her rich mellifluous voice, "Honey, Ella's dead; my name is Della and I'm still here." Amen to that.

INTERVIEW WITH DELLA REESE

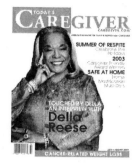

JUL / AUG 2003

Gary Barg: The whole idea of *Today's Caregiver* is to inform, educate and motivate and let the caregiver know that they are part of the solution. When I found out that you were involved with Faith in Action, I thought, "Now, there is someone who is just a living example of being part of the solution."

Della Reese: The thing I like about Faith in Action, Gary, is that people do not know that we are all a part of the solution, you see. This is an opportunity for them to find this out. A lot of people want to help, but they do not know how. The thing is, what can one person do? Well, this is what you can do. You do not have to give up your job. You do not have to give up your family. If you have one hour, you can take somebody to pick up their prescription. If you have a couple of hours, you can take somebody something to eat. You could fix somebody something to eat. You could drive somebody to a senior citizens' center so that they could be with people who think like they think and remember the things they remember.

That is so important, to be with somebody who remembers what you remember. You see, as you get older, the things that are of the day are not necessarily the things that are important to you. The things that you have been through and that you have lived through are the things that are important. For the people who live alone because their family is in another town or they do not have any family, maybe the only people they talk to are the mailman or the lady at the checkout counter of the supermarket.

They do not have anybody to come and spend time with them. I have gotten so many letters about that. I have gotten so many letters about the people being trapped in their houses because they have nobody to come and get them and take them out, and how much *Touched by an Angel* meant to them because at least once a week, somebody was saying, "God cares about you." Well, with Faith in Action, you have somebody there every day telling you that, you see.

Gary: You are saying the Faith in Action volunteers are angels.

Della: Absolutely. Most people want to do good things. Most people want to help. They just do not know how to help. We have been so disillusioned by the people who raise money and say that they go for things that help people. We find out later that it went into somebody's pocket. We do not know who to trust; but with Faith in Action, you are doing it yourself. You see it being done. You know that she got help to pick up her prescription because you took her.

Gary: I know that you have gotten bushels of mail and email and people stop you on the street talking about how *Touched by an Angel* has touched them. Have you heard specifically from family caregivers how your messages have helped them?

Della: Believe it or not, I have heard from all kinds of people. For an example, one day I was on a plane. I had a

6:00 a.m. call. I was on the 10:15 p.m. plane. I had been working all day long. I just wanted to take a nap so that I would be friendly to my husband when I landed in Los Angeles. That is all I wanted to do. This lady comes through. I was sitting in first class, but in the last seat before you go into coach. She saw me and said, "Oh, I want to thank you because your show saved my life." As I said, I was not in the greatest mood in the world. She seemed to sense that. She said, "No, I am serious. Your show saved my life." There was a line of people behind her trying to get on the plane. She did not even care. I said, "How did the show save your life?"

She said, "My husband was 26 years old. He just died. There was nothing wrong with him. There was no way for me to expect that he was going to die. I have two children. I did not know how to handle it myself, so I really did not know what to say to my children that their father was not there any more. I do not know how I ended up in the living room, but when I did, the television was on. It was *Touched by an Angel*. It was a show about a man who was dying. He was happy. He so reminded me of my husband. His family was standing around the bed. They were happy and singing. Then an angel came and got him and took him. I just adjusted to it. I was able to speak to my children about it because I knew my husband was the kind of man that wherever he was, he was happy."

Gary: That is beautiful. I believe that.

Della: I believed it, too. I believe there was no reason for her to stand there in that aisle with all those people grumbling behind her and lie.

Gary: You know, what I find consistently with family caregivers is that spirituality and religion, even if they were not religious or spiritual before, become a real keystone in their life. Every time they email me or I see them at conferences, maybe nine times out of 10, there is something about what they go through with an ill loved one that brings out the absolute best in them.

Della: Absolutely. You have to dig deep into yourself and stop being so concerned about yourself. To be a good caregiver, you have to give just that, give of yourself. You find that you are no longer so concerned with your little gripes and things. You are involved in making this person you are caring for more comfortable and happy. It is very good for you. I think it is a good thing.

Gary: So caregiving brings us back to being a community, wherever we happen to live.

Della: You know, all these machines have separated us. There was a time when it was the grandmother's job to take care of the children. The mother took care of the grandmother. There was somebody there to care. When the grandmother got old enough, they took care of her in the house so that they were there with her, but we have separated everything. We got a computer, a television and all those things that isolate us from each other. We do not have that. This is the way to bring us back to the community.

Gary: You are in a unique position as a spiritual leader and someone who has been a family caregiver. You are somebody that family caregivers reach out to. Have you come up with any advice that you would like everybody in our caregiving audience to take to heart?

Della: Well, I think the advice has already been given. One of the things is give and it shall be given to you, pressed down, shaken together and running over. It is better to give than it is to receive. You see, those sound like clichés, but they are really true. People just need somebody to say, "Come on. Let me show you. Just give this time right here and see how you feel about it."

Gary: Let me let you know that you belong. What you and your family are going through, so many other people are trying to reach out and help you, even if it is just a case of holding your hand and listening to you talk.

Della: Whatever it is, I have time for you. Instead of watching the soaps, I have time for you. Take this time right here. Let us go and sit in the park. When was the last time you fed a pigeon? Come on. Let us go to the zoo or the movies. Let us just ride around and see what is going on. When was the last time you have been shopping? Let us go look in the stores. It is not about money. It is about my caring to spend some time with you, you see. You need that. Everybody needs that. I know I need it.

INTERVIEW WITH HUGH DOWNS

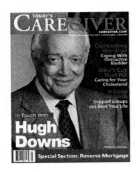

JUL / AUG 2007

Gary Barg: Tell me about the caregiving project of the ILC (International Longevity Center).

Hugh Downs: The goal of the ILC is to change the thinking of humans, particularly a lot of the Western society which is riddled with that "Pepsi generation" mentality, with the accent on youth, which really neglects and goes against older people just because they are older people; and this is still true to a large extent. I admire the ILC because it's on top of all these goals and trends and is trying to lead the world toward enlightenment; not merely for humanitarian reasons and fairness, but for the sake of civilization.

There've been cultures that have been wise enough to capture the wisdom of their elders, particularly in places such as Nepal where my son was for many years. When I went to visit him in there, the Nepalese have a custom that I thought was very interesting. We have euphemisms for "old" because "old" is supposed to be bad in our culture, so we invent words like "senior citizens" so that it will not be taken as an insult. In Nepal, the first thing they ask you when they meet you is, "How old are you?" and you answer with an apologetic response, "Well, I'm 50." Their proper and polite response is, "Well don't feel bad; you're getting there." It's just the opposite of what we do, because we like to compliment someone by saying, "You don't look that old."

Gary: I wanted to ask you about your book, *Letters to a Great-Grandson*, because to me, that's what caregiving is really about. You share your advice, your wisdom, with the generations coming after you, and you share advice about their decades yet to come. I also think as caregivers, we teach our kids everything by example, including how they watch us care for our elders.

Hugh: You're absolutely right; that's an interesting point. It helps them to grow up with the right attitude. This whole idea of how children are brought up and how they see what their parents and elders are doing makes an enormous difference because they tend to imitate. Like with abuse, which runs down chains of generations if it's left unchecked. I think the opposite is true if a person has developed empathy and has an attitude of helpfulness to their fellow people; that's going to rub off on children who are exposed to it.

Gary: I don't think I've ever heard a better comment on caregiving than a quote attributed to you, "A happy person is not a person in a certain set of circumstances, but rather a person with a certain set of attitudes."

Hugh: Isn't that true? I'm sure we both have known people who had no physical problems, no pain, who were really unhappy; and yet I've known people who have had the most horrendous kinds of health difficulties, but remain happy inside. So, it has to be a question of attitude. A favorite example of mine of how to look at things is a supposedly true story about Daniel Boone. When in his old age, he was being interviewed by a newspaper guy who asked him if he had ever been lost in the wilderness.

Boone thought for a moment and then said, "No, I was never lost. Once I was uncertain of my position for four days, but I was never lost." So, you're not lost unless you think you're lost. It's really a matter of attitude.

Gary: It doesn't matter what city we are in when we host the Fearless Caregiver Conferences across the country; one of the things that seems to be endemic to all of the events is that there will be people coming in with attitudes like "I'm handling this" and "I'm looking for information" and then there are some people coming in with a different attitude altogether. It seems that the differentiator in what they get out of the day is always their attitude.

Hugh: It really is. There's a wonderful thing I ran across a few years ago. There were these three guys in a vast field and they were all moving heavy stones. The first guy the interviewer came to he asked what he was doing, and he said, "I'm toting rocks" and he was very unhappy. The second guy went about with a more business-like attitude and when he was asked what he was doing, he said, "I'm putting up a wall." The third guy was ecstatic and happy and energetic and when he was asked what he was doing, he answered, "I am building a cathedral." Now, the big question, is how do you engender that attitude? And how does a person escape from the drudgery of all the things that come without having a proper attitude? That's a bigger problem.

Gary: I really love the title to another one of your books, *Thirty Dirty Lies about Old Age*. I know you wrote that in 1979, but what are some of those thirty dirty lies caregivers should know about today?

Hugh: A caregiver who is tactless could do a bad thing to people by exuding an attitude that is discouraging. You don't need discouragement during any time in life, but particularly when you've accumulated a lot of years. When I was doing that PBS special on aging, I was really getting fed up with so much of the prejudice and what it promoted, like "You can't teach an old dog new tricks," which isn't true, and that "You can't do anything about growing old," which may be true chronologically, but you can do something about your condition by modifying risks like quitting smoking or getting your diet under control. Another one that bothers me is that "The aged are past their prime." What is prime? Prime, in the form of wisdom, may not come for many, many decades, so this whole thing about aging and being past your prime is nonsense.

Another misconception is that "All older people want to be young." I don't particularly want to be younger than what I am, but what I would like, and it is nonsense, is a 35-year-old body and an 86-year-old outlook on wisdom, but it's not in the cards for anybody just yet. The other horrid attitude is that "Old age is an illness." That's an awful attitude to have because it's just the opposite. Our culture tends to put old age in the same basket with decrepitude and impairment, and it's just the opposite. The longer a person stays alive, the more of a triumph that person is over the forces that are constantly trying to do us in from the crib, through our prime, and into our old age. So, it's just the opposite of being an illness or a disorder.

Gary: I wish we could get the healthcare community to stop saying, "Oh, it is just old age."

Hugh: Remember in Dr. Butler's (former president and CEO of the ILC and Professor of Geriatrics and Adult Development at Mount Sinai Medical Center) book, *Why Survive?*, which is still one of the great books of all time, he had the example of the fellow who was 102 and went to the doctor because he had a bad pain in his right knee? The doctor made some therapeutic recommendation, but ended the session as doctors often do by saying, "But don't expect too much; after all, at your age ..." and the older fellow interjected, "Doctor, my other knee is also 102, and it doesn't hurt me." I thought it was a great example of how one should think about that.

Gary: Is there one specific piece of advice you'd like to leave family caregivers with who are reading this?

Hugh: My advice to them, if they want to be effective in what they are doing, is to exercise all their empathetic talents and feelings so that they really do care about the person that they are taking care of. Secondly, is to be sure that they never do anything that destroys hope. Whatever the person's need is that you're taking care of, help them nurture hope. Above all, see to it that they have what they need for comfort, because the alleviation of suffering is everything; and as I said earlier, there are people who are suffering without a lot of physical pain, and then there are those who are tolerating considerable pain and are not suffering with it. The alleviation of suffering should be the whole goal of every doctor, every nurse, every psychiatrist, and every caregiver. Caregivers can help with this greatly, I think, because they are close to the people a lot of the time, and they can help sustain hope.

INTERVIEW WITH ED ASNER

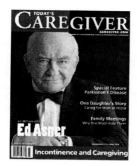

SEPT / OCT 2008

Gary Barg: I am a real fan of your work with the Humane Society of the United States and trying to promote the idea of pet trusts.

Ed Asner: Well, I think it is cruel not to make plans for what happens to your pets when you die. When I was married, we had three kids. We had a vast menagerie of animals: three big dogs, four or five cats, turtles, fish, birds, you name it. We even had a lab rat that got loose. And it filled our lives and it was a wonderful glue to bind us together. Then eventually my wife and I divorced and for 26 years I went without an animal. I had 26 years without a cat in my life and it is night and day for me to have them in my life now.

Gary: Animals are so very important. I have a friend, Dr. Bill Thomas, who created the Eden Alternative, and that is where there is a whole plan in place for facilities to actually incorporate pets and plants; it brings back people from the edge because now they have something to love and something to take care of.

Ed: That is lovely. That is really lovely.

Gary: In another light, I know you were involved in the elder abuse prevention video called "Saving Our Parents." I thought your first words in that really hit home. You said "If you do not care for your senior loved ones, people with less than loving intentions will be more than happy to lend a hand." And I think that nothing is truer and nothing is sadder.

Ed: Well, yes.

Gary: I wonder if you have thought about how someone can protect themselves and their loved ones from all the scams and the frauds and the Internet crimes and identity thefts out there.

Ed: Observation of an elder parent will help you find out just what is going on. Talk with them about what they are involved in. And exercise greater caution and care about checking out their mail and checking out what they are responding to and even checking out phone messages. We do not do enough butting in on parents, within reason. I know I am so annoyed that in our family of five kids, none of us ever really sat our old man down or the old lady and asked what was it like, what did you do? And of my mother in particular: How she lived before she came from Russia and the Ukraine. We never discussed that.

Gary: I agree with you. My dad, who passed away about 12 years ago, would be 78 now, and when he became ill, I did not want to make him feel that I am talking about the end of his life; yet it could have been a great experience to tape a conversation with him. I think that it is a shame for the next generations to lose that connectivity. How would you ask your kids to sit down and have this conversation with you?

Ed: My wonderful secretary bought a book which leads the way in what questions to ask. And unfortunately, every time she asked me a question, I went off for a half hour responding and it became an enormous drag to listen. And that is what you have got to expect. So I would advise you to buy one of these books. They are filled with very good questions to stimulate the memory.

Gary: I think it is good because it does stimulate their memory and makes them think about things that may be lost after they are gone; and of course, it connects us to our past.

Ed: And it engenders in the talker the fact that, done well enough and done fully enough, death will not obliterate them. I think that is a very satisfying thing to have. It is just that we do not take the time.

Gary: I think we do not take the time and like you and I, we do not think about it until after it is too late.

Ed: There was an organization and they got my mother's youngest sister on audio and videotape. It may not be the most electric piece of video done, but it is there. It is there to go back to whenever we want.

Gary: It means something to your family.

Ed: Yes.

Gary: You are obviously still very active in your career and your life. I am wondering if you have any recommendations for caregivers about helping their aging parents stay healthy, involved, active.

Ed: To the best of your ability, you need to order them

about, making plans with them; and get them in the habit of getting up and about and out, checking to be sure what fascinates them at this point in time.

Gary: I think you are right. We do not stay involved enough. We do not nudge enough.

Ed: Yes, and sometimes they are going to resist. Hey, I would resist. My kids found a way to tell me: "You are going to get off your butt and you are going to go to this place with me." And stewing in the idea a couple times a week can make a big difference. Finally, it becomes a habit and they start asking you: "Aren't you coming by to pick me up?"

Gary: What would you consider the one most important piece of advice you can share with a family caregiver?

Ed: I have a friend. For years, he and his wife took care of an old Hungarian seamstress and the stories they got from her: the romances, and affairs, and the mighty that she had known made their caregiving a very cheap price to pay. So, mine that mother lode of history and you are bound to get rewarded.

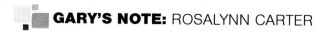

GARY'S NOTE: ROSALYNN CARTER

The first time I met Former First Lady Rosalynn Carter was in 1996 at an event in Miami. I was given the honor of introducing her to the audience of family caregivers. *Today's Caregiver* magazine had just celebrated its first anniversary and there were not many people in the world talking about the needs of family caregivers. Among the few pioneers who were around when we launched the magazine was, in fact, Mrs. Carter since the Rosalynn Carter Institute had been founded 14 years earlier.

I met with her backstage and was at once struck by her grace as well as her striking blue eyes. She was sipping tea as she was battling a sore throat which made it difficult for her to talk. Yet, I do remember her presence and power during her speech; I don't think the audience knew at all how much every word hurt her to speak. Every time I talk with her, I remember to thank her for myself and everyone who ever gives a speech about caregiving since we all steal these lines from her book *Helping Yourself Help Others:* "There are only four kinds of people in the world – those who have been caregivers, those who are currently caregivers, those who will be caregivers and those who will need caregivers..." Truer words have never been spoken.

INTERVIEW WITH ROSALYNN CARTER

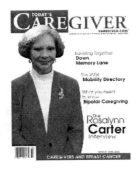

MAR / APR 2004

Gary Barg: How did you get involved in helping caregivers?

Rosalynn Carter: I got into helping caregivers because of my mental health work. I had worked with families who had a mentally ill family member, and I knew how hard it was for the families. So many times, those illnesses come on suddenly, and families see the first mental health professional in an emergency room. The families don't have any idea of what to do or where to go, so when we came home from the White House, I decided I could do something for them.

We started working with those who were caring for mentally ill family members. The idea quickly spread because in our community, everybody knows everybody, and so we knew who in the community was a caregiver. Our first session was on burnout, and there were people who were caring for frail-elderly or physically ill family members who wanted to come, so even before our first, big conference, it had expanded to caring for people across the board of need.

Gary: Did you also have a personal reason for organizing this kind of help for caregivers?

Rosalynn: I've been a caregiver for a good part of my life. My father died when I was thirteen, and I am the oldest of four children, so I helped my mother. One of my main responsibilities was to help her with the smaller children, but I also helped her with my father. The following year, her mother died, and my mother was the only child, so my grandfather came to live with us; he was 70 and lived to be 95. I helped with him as well. My mother worked at the post office and the postmaster gave her hours in the morning and hours in the afternoon so that she could go home for lunch and take care of him. But I helped with him when she needed to go to work.

Also, since we've come home from the White House, all of Jimmy's family members have died from cancer ... his mother, his brother, and his two sisters ... his whole immediate family, and I've watched that process, too, so I have the personal experience that makes me value the caregivers.

Gary: Do you have one specific take-home lesson from all your caregiving experience?

Rosalynn: What we've learned at the Rosalynn Carter Institute is if you don't learn to care for yourself, then you're not going to be able to be the best caregiver that you can be for the one who is ill. That was the book I wrote, *Helping Yourself Help Others.*

Gary: That's a great book and I have a favorite quote from it, "There are only four kinds of people in the world: those who have been caregivers, those who are currently caregivers, those who will be caregivers and those who will need caregivers." How did that phrase come about and did you know that it would have such an impact?

Rosalynn: No, I didn't. When I began working with the university, which was a public college back then, the man who was the head of the institute was also the head of the psychology department. He was a psychologist and had cared for his mother and father for a long time by himself. I don't even think they lived in the same community with him, but he really had a tough time trying to do what he was doing and also care for his mother and father. He was the one who actually gave me that quote.

Gary: How can people help support your work at the Rosalynn Carter Institute?

Rosalynn: Right now we're raising an endowment so that it can go on after I'm no longer able to raise money for it. It's the only university-based caregiving center, which is kind of nice, and we raise money; but we do receive grants from Johnson & Johnson and from the Area Agency on Aging.

Gary: Do you have any advice for family caregivers?

Rosalynn: The best advice I think I can give them is to leave some time for themselves. They have to have some escape from the caregiving duties. Take some time, even if you can't get away totally. I know one woman whose mother was sick, and couldn't get out, so she had to be taken care of all the time. Her mother wanted to see what her flowers looked like in the garden, so the woman began photographing the roses, other flowers and the trees so her mother could see the change of seasons. She got so good, she now has a photography business in her home.

Even if it's just gardening, or walking around the house, or reading a good book, people need something to take their mind off of their duty. A lot of people don't like to say that they have a duty or a burden when it comes to caregiving, because there are rewards. I think that everybody feels some reward. There was a woman who said that she got so upset with her father at times, that she felt like running away. She said that one day, she did run away; she left him in his wheelchair and checked into a hotel downtown. She stayed for only a few hours because she felt so guilty. When she returned home, he was still in his wheelchair just where she had left him.

People just need some outlet. One thing that people can do is to look up the Rosalynn Carter Institute on the Internet (www.rosalynncarter.org) and see what we're doing, and send us messages for advice. People also need to know that there is help in the community, and we can help caregivers locate organizations and support groups.

INTERVIEW WITH JOY & EVE BEHAR

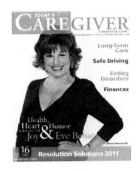

JAN / FEB 2011

Gary Barg: How has heart disease affected your family?

Joy Behar: I am the recipient of a gene, I think possibly, because my mother had her first heart attack when she was 50 years old. I have an uncle who is her brother who had a heart attack and died at the age of 58, a sudden heart attack. Both my grandparents on my mother's side died of heart attacks. So, there you have it. It is not a pretty picture.

Gary: What do women need to know about the risks of having sudden heart attacks and what should they do if they think they are experiencing one?

Joy: Well, I think it is sort of logical in a way. If you feel like you are having a heart attack, you should call 911 immediately.

Gary: My grandmother also passed without warning from a heart attack at the age of 65, in the 60s, and my mom has long been aware of her own possible heart issues. I was wondering what I should tell my nieces, who are both in their 20s, about what their possible risk is and what they might need to do to pay attention to their own heart health.

Joy: At that age, prevention is really where it's at, so exercise and eat well.

Eve: Keep the weight down and tell them not to smoke. That is elementary to say you do not smoke at that age. A lot of girls in that age bracket want to stay skinny and they think by smoking they will not get fat, but they could also kill themselves.

Joy: That is a good point for these young girls.

Eve: And also women, as they age, they get busier and busier, and they start taking care of other people more than themselves. So that is something you could say to them is you really need to take care of yourself first, and then you will be able to take care of everybody else. I am pregnant now and I am going to be a new mom, so that is on my mind that I have to take care of myself so I can take care of my baby.

Joy: Right, exactly, and young women, like your nieces, they can also talk to their moms to start taking their heart health seriously. Maybe they are just in their 20s so they do not have kids yet necessarily. They are just working on their own careers, but their moms are right at the age where they could suffer a heart attack. So young women should be talking to their mothers. Talk to your doctor and in case you have a heart attack or you think you are having a heart attack, call 911 and pop an aspirin.

Gary: Joy, I would like to say thank you for your children's book *Sheetzucacapoopoo: My Kind of Dog*. Now that is another book I have to buy since my tiny two-foot tan tyrant is taking up 90 percent of my chair. I bring my dog to work every day, so I think the thing that keeps me from having heart attacks is having him around all day.

Eve: That is true. We have pets and we love them and they add a lot of joy and keep your stress level down; they've proven that.

Joy: Yes. That is important, and laughing and having fun.

Gary: What would be the one most important piece of advice you can offer to a family caregiver?

Joy: Go to your doctor. Make sure that you know if you are at risk for a heart attack. It is very, very important. Take care of yourself, exercise, walk, eat the right things, do not smoke, all the stuff that we all know already that people take for granted. Women think they are already doing everything. They are not; and get your cholesterol checked every year. Get an EKG. There are so many things you can do. Know your risk; be prepared. Those are the words. It is like the Boy Scouts. Be prepared, but know your risks.

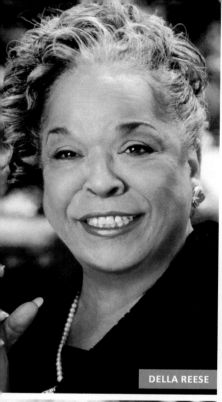

DELLA REESE

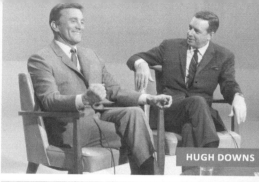

HUGH DOWNS

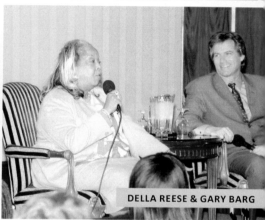

DELLA REESE & GARY BARG

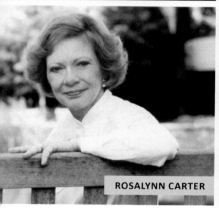

ROSALYNN CARTER

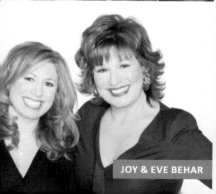

JOY & EVE BEHAR

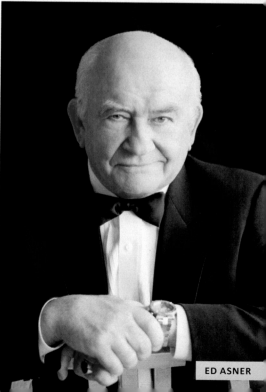

ED ASNER

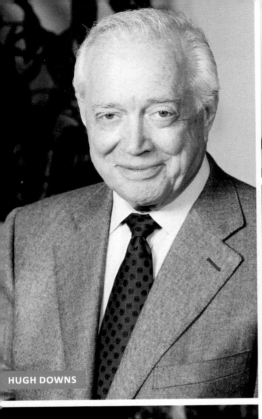

HUGH DOWNS

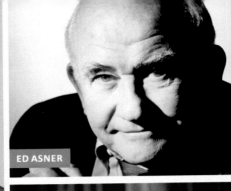

ED ASNER

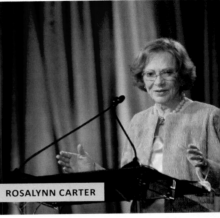

ROSALYNN CARTER

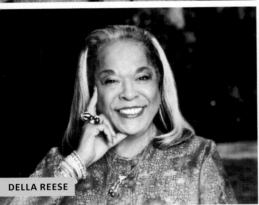

DELLA REESE

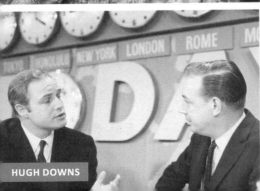

HUGH DOWNS

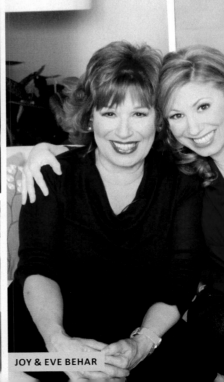

JOY & EVE BEHAR

Caring for
PARENTS

*Do not lose your sense of humor. My grandmother lived with
my parents for the last five years of her life. There's nothing
greater than being able to take care of an elder in those final
years. I think my mother and father being able to laugh at some
of the crazy, embarrassing things that were happening got them
through some tough, tough patches.*

— Jane Kaczmarek

GARY'S NOTE: DEBBIE REYNOLDS

I think I never learned more about stage presence than in the two days I spent with Debbie Reynolds at the Phoenix and Cleveland Fearless Caregiver Conferences. When I first met her backstage, she was extremely pleasant, but quite low-key. Once I introduced her to the audience of family caregivers, it was obvious why she is such a star. Once she took to the stage, she immediately transformed from a quiet and shy lady to an incredible dynamo with stars shooting out every pore. The lesson: keep the energy stored for those times when you are on stage and then give them all you've got. Also, it was impressive to hear her answer every personal question asked of her by the family caregivers openly and honestly, without hesitation. Her presence reminded me that when you have 400 family caregivers and one celebrity caregiver together in a room, you actually have 401 family caregivers.

INTERVIEW WITH DEBBIE REYNOLDS

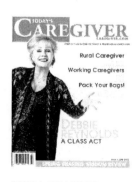

MAY / JUN 2003

Gary Barg: You have a unique approach to talking about caregiving. Can you tell me a little about that?

Debbie Reynolds: I try to get the point across without being too dead-serious. It is such a difficult subject, and it's life. Life is not a bowl of cherries; because if it were, why am I feeling in the pits? My family has a history of longevity; my mom lived to be 82 and my daddy,

83. We all have caregiving situations. Every generation has to take care of the next generation, or not and not care at all. I don't think "we" as a people feel this way, because most of us want to take care of our loved ones. Not everybody gets to live well towards the end. Because people are living longer, you either have to take them into your home or find a place for them. This type of decision-making can either be life threatening or life making.

Gary: What is your personal experience with caregiving?

Debbie: My grandmother lived with my mom and Daddy until she went blind, and then my mother became critically ill with a bad heart. My mother started having heart conditions when she was 39, so I've been a caregiver since I was 14. Mother became very ill and we had to put my grandmother with her other children, who were also very good to her. All this time, my grandmother suffered from osteoporosis. My family seems to weather the storms, but they have a lot of health problems that still exist today. I am a caregiver for my brother who is only 62, and we still live together. This is why I've been so involved with all these causes. When breast cancer awareness first came out, I was one of the first spokespersons for a test to detect that. When osteoporosis awareness came out, I became a spokesperson to take tests for this as well. And now we have the problem of incontinence, or over-active bladder, which I guess just sounds nicer. My mother and father both had it, and it was the most embarrassing problem for them to overcome. In fact, they never did overcome it; we just had to deal with it because at that time, there was no help. I went to the doctors about it, but there was no pill, there was nothing. So when I was asked to represent a drug for incontinence, I said "Yes!" I was so happy to do it because I did not have that help when my parents really needed it. It was especially difficult for my father.

Gary: I was wondering what advice you would have for families who may be just beginning to deal with the issue of incontinence.

Debbie: They have to run, not walk, to the doctor. We know that the doctors know of a couple different pharmaceutical companies that have a pill that can be given to the patient and eliminate the incontinence; not all together, but at least where it can be controlled for long periods of hours, where they can actually function and be social and active again; not hide out in their room and not be embarrassed to death. The problem is, they lose their will to go out because they can't go out, because they have to time when to go out, and they don't know when they're going to have this problem. So, they must talk to their doctor. There are at least 17 million people who suffer from this, and that's only in this country.

Gary: How did your parents deal with the problem?

Debbie: I had to put them in diapers. My father wouldn't discuss it, however. I was the only one he would allow to change his diapers. Otherwise, he would remain in it, and this was impossible, and so it became extremely hard to care for him. My mother finally put him in a home against all of my wishes, but he did do better there because they had a male nurse. But these are extreme measures. I always advise to try homecare if possible, if you have the money, if it is a financial possibility to keep them at home, if you can convert a room, because they demand so little, really. Of course, that's not true of some personalities, if dementia is involved, because there are all these levels of illnesses.

Gary: Caregivers seem to buzz about you days after you have spoken at an event. What do they say to you with regard to their personal stories?

Debbie: The families ask me what to do, especially about Alzheimer's disease because that's what my father had, along with the incontinence. Poor Daddy, he really got it all at the end. It was difficult to nurse him because he didn't want to be nursed. He was part Cherokee, and he just wanted to be taken out to the desert. That's what he kept telling me. "Look," he would say, "just take me out to the desert, put a blanket over me, and life will just go." That's an impossibility to do, but he thought that was the ideal way to go—ashes to ashes, dust to dust.

Gary: I'm honored to spend some time with you. I think you're helping a whole lot of families out there as you go around sharing your message with them.

Debbie: Well, we try. Sometimes you don't get through to people. Not every talk show wants to discuss this. It's sad to me that they don't want to recognize this problem. They want me to just come on and talk about *Singing in the Rain* and all the fun things in my life; which I do, but I try to work this in, in my own sneaky way.

INTERVIEW WITH ROB LOWE

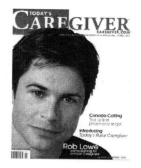

JAN / FEB 2003

Gary Barg: You are working to inform people about the negative side effects of chemotherapy. With your Dad, the side effects threw your family for a loop. Nobody told you about it beforehand?

Rob Lowe: Cancer doesn't play favorites, and it's sort of the great equalizer. Anyone fighting cancer, or anyone living with or loving someone fighting cancer—it's just the same for me as anybody else. We all want new information, we all want strength and hope. We were aware of hair loss, nausea, bloating, and all those things you usually associate with chemo, but we didn't know that infection is a very common side effect, and potentially a life-threatening one. Knowing would have made a big difference to us going in, because my dad's chemo was stopped when his count was down and he'd gotten an infection. Luckily, it wasn't as bad for him as it is for others. Some people have to go into the hospital. Some people have to be isolated from their families, and, unfortunately, some do die from it. So I wanted that word to get out because today, with new medicines, you can protect yourself right out the door for the most part.

Gary: I think our dads were diagnosed about the same time, '90, '91. I remember infection was a problem. They'd have to stop his chemo and then you don't get the positive effects; you have to change your chemo again.

Rob: And they really didn't have the new medicines. Yes, that's exactly what happened to my dad. As those things go, he was on the good luck side of it, but he thought he was dying when he came home and he couldn't have his chemo. Forget the logical mind; what he thought was, "They told me I can't have my chemo. I'm dying."

Gary: What would you like families to know up front when cancer is an issue?

Rob: The number one thing is to take notes and ask questions going in. Doctors are amazing, and they saved my father's life, but remember they work for you. One thing to specifically ask is, "Am I going to be at risk for infection, and if so, should I be treated for it before we begin?" Invariably, you leave the doctor's office, you drive a mile, and then you go, "Oh, I didn't ask about..." And then you don't want to call, and when you do call, you're on hold and you feel uncomfortable.

Gary: So, don't be ashamed and learn to reach out, because other people are going through this.

Rob: Oh yeah, because the old cliché is true, "Knowledge is power."

Gary: The difference between being a caregiver and not being a caregiver is that telephone call in the middle of night. What was it like for you and your family when you first found out about your father's diagnosis?

Rob: I think it's always surreal for anyone who gets that call. To make matters even more surreal, I was in Israel shooting a movie where I was playing a Navy SEAL and they were handing out gas masks. At that point, Saddam Hussein was threatening to launch biological weapons on Tel Aviv. This was right before Desert Storm, and I was in a surreal place to begin with. I remember when the phone rang, I remember the certain layout of the room, and how the sun was coming through the window, and all those details; and yet, I don't remember any of the conversation because it was too uncomfortable, sad and shocking.

Gary: That's an interesting point. For those first six months, for the caregiver, it's a total haze.

Rob: One of the most interesting things I've learned is that research shows when a patient is diagnosed, from that point on, they only retain about 10 percent of the information they are given. It makes sense logically, but it's a stunning figure.

Gary: It's true, and I like the concept that people are able to "hold hands" with other experienced cancer caregivers.

Rob: It's all based on my experience with my father. He would be very reticent to get into anything with me, or with immediate members of his family, but I would see him open up to an abject stranger in a shopping mall—someone who looked like they had also gone through chemo. There's just no substitute for talking to people who are going through what you are going through, or who have gone through it.

Gary: I saw this lovely quote of yours on the Web which says, "My grandmother, Peg Helper, had breast cancer and I watched her fight it for almost 20 years. Through it all, my grandfather was so supportive, which inspired me; every man should approach this disease with the same dignity." I thought that was a great way to talk about the challenges of male caregivers. Any advice or any points you want to make?

Rob: When talking specifically about male caregivers, it makes me think of my grandmother, and the husbands who are caring for their wives, mothers or their daughters; and I can just remember the amazing way my grandfather would just love my grandmother as a "woman," and not just as a patient. That can be really, really hard. That's really critical, because I remember when my grandmother came home with a wig, my grandfather kept telling her how beautiful she looked in her new wig… that kind of stuff, that man and woman stuff, you've got to try to keep alive.

Gary: What has stood out the most for you from your experience?

Rob: People always ask me what this has been like for me—meeting the mothers who are fighting disease while raising their kids, the fathers who still coach little league, or go into the office, the children who fight and never lose their optimism or hope—they are the real American heroes.

INTERVIEW WITH DAVID HYDE PIERCE

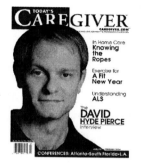

JAN / FEB 2004

Gary Barg: As a board member of the Alzheimer's Association, you must have a good understanding of the progress being made to help people with Alzheimer's and their caregivers. Do you think we're any closer to finding a cure?

David Hyde Pierce: We're always closer to getting a cure, but we're still not close enough. The researchers have been working tirelessly, and we have some of the best people in the scientific world focused on this disease; because it is such an enigma and such a tragedy on so many different levels. People for humanitarian reasons, for economic reasons, for all sorts of reasons want to find a way to slow this disease down. In fact, even more than a cure, if we could just find a way to slow it down so that people do what they used to do a hundred years ago; which is, for the most part, pass away before it ever became a problem.

Gary: Do the drugs on the market today really help slow down the progression?

David: Absolutely. The drugs that are available now affect every individual differently; some people respond more to one than others, and others respond better to a combination or drugs. There are more drugs certainly in the pipeline to help mainly with the symptoms, allowing more time for people to plan, to be with their families and to be as independent for as long as possible.

Gary: Tell me a little about the PBS television show, *Alzheimer's: the Help You Need.* You hosted this panel discussion that follows the broadcast of *The Forgetting: A Portrait of Alzheimer's.*

David: Any time you are caring for a loved one, it's difficult; especially if you are caring for a loved one with a terminal illness. But there is something so torturous about what Alzheimer's disease puts caregivers through. So on this panel, along with scientific experts, we had people who are social workers, people who are dealing with the caregiving aspect of it because that is as important as treating the one with the disease. My grandfather had it and my dad probably had it, although he had stroke-induced dementia at first; but it likely became Alzheimer's toward the end. In both cases, my grandmother who was my grandfather's caregiver and my mother who was my father's caregiver predeceased their spouses. My grandmother died of a stroke, and there's just no question that the emotional stress plus the physical stress of dealing with my grandfather, seeing his decline, and dealing with the round-the-clock supervision that he required—I'm sure it ended her life long before she would have died.

Gary: So often each caregiver thinks that they are the only one who can take care of their loved one.

David: That's something we address in the panel discussion as well. That whole concept of the airline motif, where you put on your oxygen mask first before you help someone else who needs it. If you are not taking care of yourself, how will you be able to take care of the person you love? Ultimately, you do both of yourselves a disservice.

Gary: Taking care of yourself first could be our motto at *Today's Caregiver*, but there seems to be an added guilt factor when caring for someone living with Alzheimer's.

David: Along with all of the other responsibilities of caregiving with Alzheimer's or any other dementia disorder, the person being taken care of can't be responsible for themselves; so they do things like wandering away, or leaving something on the stove and burning the house down; or they are unable to communicate what might be a very simple ailment, so you don't see it until it becomes a chronic condition. So, added to all of the burdens on the caregiver, you almost have to think for and intuit for the person you are taking care of, because they may do themselves harm inadvertently.

Gary: One of the subjects discussed in the panel discussion was, "How do you take the keys away?" How do you take the keys away?

David: Well, I'll tell you how we did it with my dad. He was in an early stage of dementia when we realized he had just enough scrapes on the car that we had not witnessed. We thought we were at the point that his independence had to become secondary to his and other people's safety.

We had a family meeting, and we knew we needed to take the keys away. What we ended up doing was we talked to his heart doctor, who had been a real confidant, and he suggested that he handle it. We brought Dad in, and my brother and I went with him. My dad was sitting on the examining table and the doctor said, "Well, George, you have a touch of Alzheimer's, so I think it's going to be better if you don't drive," and Dad gave him the keys. That did a bunch of things. First of all, it was sort of a bogus diagnosis, but it was an effective diagnosis. By using the phrase "a touch of Alzheimer's," it took the curse off of it, especially at that point in my dad's decline. He knew something was up and it somehow didn't have the same impact as saying "You have Alzheimer's disease" would. It was just a "touch," just enough that we probably should be cautious. I cannot praise this doctor enough. He knew my dad so well, that he knew he would respond to that. And afterwards, Dad confessed that he was so relieved; he didn't want to have to give up driving, but every time he got behind the wheel of the car, he was petrified.

Dad had a combination of what's called "vascular dementia" caused by a stroke after heart surgery, so there were already some peripheral vision problems that were occurring and he was getting lost. So, I would only add that someone else in that situation, the doctor might have said the same thing and he might have gotten a very different response; every case is different.

Gary: What advice do you have for family caregivers?

David: Especially with Alzheimer's, the first thing is that if you haven't gotten in touch with the Alzheimer's Association in your area, do it. By the time I joined the Alzheimer's Association, I was no longer in the position of having a family member with the disease; but you have the scars, you have the emotional wounds and the feeling of loss. The Alzheimer's Association has been an incredible source of strength, healing, and determination for me. But for someone who is actually going through it, and I have recommended it to many of my friends who are just starting out on this difficult path, just to have someone to talk to, to have a support group, to have a support group for the person with Alzheimer's, to have references, to have people who have been through this. That's the great thing about the Association; virtually everyone who is there, is there because they have seen this first-hand, and we're all just determined to wipe it out in our lifetime.

▪ **GARY'S NOTE:** LEEZA GIBBONS

I was truly thankful for Kimberly-Clark for bringing a truckload of Kleenex® to the 2004 Fort Lauderdale Fearless Caregiver Conference because we were joined by caregiver advocate and co-founder of the Leeza Gibbons Memory Foundation, Leeza Gibbons, and her father, Carlos Gibbons, Sr. After meeting Leeza's dad, I understand from whom Leeza gets her warmth, humanity and showbiz talents. Carlos, Sr. touched the soul of each and every person at the luncheon with his unscripted and poignant dedication to his wife Jean, daughter Leeza and entire family. At one point, Leeza lovingly yelled, "YALE," a reference to a joke Carlos told at the beginning of his talk relating to the quality of short speeches. I truly didn't care if he ever stopped talking. He was touching, funny and true to the spirit of every caregiver in the room. We were also honored to have in attendance Leeza's brother, Carlos, Jr. or Carl. I hope I am not hurting his standing with the South Carolina Bar by saying that he is a truly nice guy. Sister Cami stayed at home with Mom so Carlos and Carl could join us for the day.

Then, just when we thought nothing could ever move us more than Carlos' words, Leeza got up and knocked it out of the ballpark, simply by talking about her dad's love for her mother. I had three friends come up to me later and tell me that the bathrooms were filled with people trying to regain composure and fixing running mascara. And when I returned to the office later that night, I had already received a handful of emails containing the exact same words, "not a dry eye in the place."

INTERVIEW WITH LEEZA GIBBONS

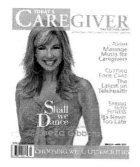

MAR / APR 2007

Gary Barg: How did your commitment to helping people with Alzheimer's disease and their caregivers get started?

Leeza Gibbons: With my grandmother, we just kind of accepted that "Granny's losing it," thinking that she was going senile; we'd kind of roll our eyes and laugh at some of her disturbing behavior. She would always make these little biscuits for us, little brown jugs she called them, best thing on earth. We would find biscuits in drawers, in cabinets, and under the bed. She kind of laughed it off, but that's the first time I remember recognizing it in my grandmother. And then I saw what happened, the dynamic between my mother and her sister, who were conflicted about Granny's care. So you would think that I would have more awareness, and that I'd have my eyes wide-open when it came to my own mother, but I didn't; none of us in the family did. You'd think that we'd be more educated, more aware, and more perceptive; but when we began seeing Mom get disoriented and repeat herself and misplace things, and her personality began to change, we thought she was drinking.

Gary: What was your first thought?

Leeza: I got on the phone with my brother and sister and said, "Look, we're going to have to have an intervention; we're going to have to get her to Betty Ford." Truly, not that alcoholism is ever simple, and it is a disease that is brutal; but many times, I rewind that conversation and think how different it would be if she were an alcoholic. We could treat her and she could be part of it. But we're thankful every day that my very strong mother of generous spirit had the foresight to prevent us, as siblings, from bickering because she was very clear about what she wanted for her care. She was specific to the point that my brother is very uncomfortable with the charge of "Please talk about it" and "Please do what you can in your own lives to be advocates. That's the best way you can honor me."

Gary: Then you feel that communicating right upfront is a way for a person living with Alzheimer's to have some say in their care, past the point when they are able to express their desires?

Leeza: It was very empowering for Mom. Once she named it and claimed it and could stop covering, Dad could stop making excuses. She had a reason for the behavior, and she could come from a position of power. It's ironic that that's the process, but I think that often times, you do feel freer just knowing what it is and being able to be upfront with people.

Gary: Really what you're saying is that isolating yourself as a caregiver doesn't help you and it doesn't help your loved one.

Leeza: I think there's so much danger in that. Depression is obviously the byproduct of all of these diseases and if you drink, if you overeat, if you become a recluse, however it is that you manifest that, all of those things are potentially so dangerous to your own health that you can't be of any service to the one that you want to provide for.

Gary: One of the things I'm especially impressed with regarding the Leeza Gibbons Foundation is that you really do take the caregiver's needs to heart. I love the offsite Jean and Carlos Gibbons Family Workshops. Could you explain this a little bit?

Leeza: We were hoping that we could create a safe haven where people feel comfortable just to come in and be heard. Erasing the stigma was a big motivating factor for us, but also helping people find answers, helping them uncover the resources that are out there. Helping to make the appointments, helping them to feel that they are a part of, should they choose to be, the greater mission towards the cure.

Gary: Do you have any advice for families if they think someone is showing the first signs of a memory disorder?

Leeza: I would think the first thing to do would be to find a safe way, within your own family, to go through a checklist with your loved one, just to see if there's reason to be concerned. Then take that information to their primary care physician and begin to ask the questions. I would really encourage families to be proactive and once they suspect they are dealing with a memory disorder, make it known and ask the physician to do a cognitive test.

Gary: Sometimes you have to demand it. Sometimes a physician, especially if they have been a longtime physician and family friend, doesn't want to see it either.

Leeza: If there's a trusted physician that has a relationship with your loved one, you want to honor that; but ask that person for a referral to a specialist, because I do think that valuable time is wasted while people respect their comfort zones for very long. I do think that knowledge is power, and I do think the sooner the family begins the emotional process and the physical process of navigating down this path, the better. I can't think of a single advantage of waiting. People's wishes are then not honored, or not known. The nuts and bolts of the disease are pretty overwhelming, so early diagnosis allows families to look seriously at durable powers of attorney, and wills and all those other things we know so well. Those are hard things, I think, especially for children to discuss with their parents.

Gary: One thing that I've actually committed to memory from the information you sent, and I love this phrase, "realistic and coordinated national strategy to finding a cure." That should be a mantra. There hasn't been anything this coordinated or maybe even this realistic, that addresses all aspects of looking for a cure.

Leeza: Part of what we want to do with the foundation is to "gather up." If it's blood samples, if it's volunteers for protocols, if it's funding, or grants and studies, getting patients into research, providing data with minority groups which have been very underrepresented—we want to do all of those things, and want to escalate the time with which that information gets through the pipeline. Clearly, we're not naïve and we're not fear-based; we're very hopeful. We avail ourselves of all the research, we do all the things that are known at this point that can be done with lifestyle and diet and exercise, nutritional supplements. I thank God every night, and put at the top of my list all the people who are looking for cures. I hope that it's not just to pacify my own fears because I think that it is a real place to come from—to believe that, while there might not be cure soon, there will be treatment, there will be vaccines. You have to hang onto that.

INTERVIEW WITH MARIA SHRIVER

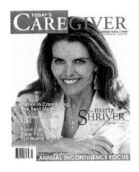

SEPT / OCT 2004

Gary Barg: Was there a moment when you first knew that your father was living with Alzheimer's disease?

Maria Shriver: I didn't have a specific moment in time. I think, like anybody in this situation, as your parents get older, you become more aware that certain things aren't the way they used to be. When he was diagnosed with Alzheimer's, we just all came together and said, "Okay, what do we do, how do we handle this the best way we can, how do we handle this as a family, how do we support Dad the best we can?" The important thing to realize is that no two cases are alike, so no two families travel the same road; what is right for one family may not be right for the other, and that doesn't mean that one is better or worse than the other.

Gary: You've had so many interesting jobs and careers, first of all as a mother, then as a First Lady, and as a reporter and anchor, how does your father's illness fit in your daily life?

Maria: Your family, whether it's your children, your spouse, your parents, your siblings, is always on your mind. I think that as with all women, I just try to navigate each day the best I can. Right now, I'm visiting my parents, so it's been parent-intensive. You ask for God's grace and for His help. I try to move forward, and the role of First Lady or as reporter doesn't really tie into my day-to-day life. I try to be a reporter at all times to learn what I can, and talk to as many people as I can when I'm given an assignment about it (Alzheimer's); but other than that, you just go through your life trying to do the best you can, doing it elegantly, and with grace and dignity. That's my motto.

Gary: What kind of response have you gotten to the publication of *What's Happening to Grandpa?*

Maria: It's been on the New York Times Bestseller's List, which was a goal of mine, so I'm very happy about that, and I get extraordinary responses. I had a man who came up to me today, not but an hour ago, and told me that he had put his mother into assisted living and that she has Alzheimer's. He started to cry and said that this book meant everything to him, and he's in his 50s. So I'm getting reactions from kids, from parents and from spouses. It has been truly wonderful and I think it's one of those books that will be there for many of the other families that will have to deal with this issue.

Gary: So the book became therapy for you, too?

Maria: Yeah, absolutely, and I hope that it will be a friend to and helpful for millions of other people.

Gary: One thing I like in particular is that it is very accessible, allowing a new caregiver to explain to a child what is going on with the disease.

Maria: Yes, I hope that it is, because you must explain to your children, and to your children's children. This is my public service for Alzheimer's, to try and spare some people from, "Oh my gosh, how do I explain this?" So now, there's a book.

Gary: How should someone navigate their way as a caregiver of someone living with Alzheimer's disease?

Maria: I think that every family deals with it in different ways, and I think it's important that every family know that they are doing the best they can, and that what's right for them is right for them, and not to judge, "Well this person was able to stay at home and care for their loved one and I'm unable to do this, so I must be bad." I think we need to be very conscious of not doing that to people, and that we all figure out that everyone develops their caregiving situation the best way that they can for their family.

Gary: So by sharing your experience, you can help other people who are going through a similar thing.

Maria: As in anything, you get strength from other people who have been through it, you learn from other people; you're constantly learning because no two days are ever alike and the disease is constantly changing, so you have to be flexible, to really live in the moment and roll with it. I have great respect for people who are caregivers and who either do that in an assisted living home, or who do it in their own home. I think that it is emotionally tough, tough work. I think caregivers are like teachers. They're in there all the time working, and are required to have creativity, patience, emotional strength, and physical strength; they have my utmost respect.

Gary: One of the first things I find caregivers doing is beating themselves up over the things they can't do, what they can't fix, and I say, "You have more on your plate, and you handle more on a daily basis than any major CEO of any company I've ever met."

Maria: Right, and I think it's important to continue lauding people in that profession. Keep trying to understand the person who has Alzheimer's, and to keep growing with it. There are always great lessons in all of this, so you keep trying to learn, and you keep trying to evolve, even if you're not the primary caregiver.

Gary: What are some suggestions you have for caregivers?

Maria: A lot of this is just life's lessons. You have to try and take care of yourself, especially if you have to take care of someone else. People who are caregivers, who are on the frontlines, are the experts; and they need to remember that they may not necessarily have to speak to someone else if what they are doing is working well for them.

INTERVIEW WITH JOAN LUNDEN

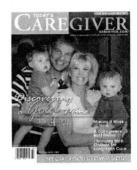

JUL / AUG 2005

Gary Barg: As a family caregiver, I have to thank you for your message of the importance of positive attitudes. One of your quotes that I really like is, "We can't stop changes from occurring, but we can control how we react to them." What an important lesson for family caregivers.

Joan Lunden: The most important thing to understand is the concept that we actually have the ability to not react, and I truly believe that most people don't think that way. People think that when something happens, they must react in a fashion that then determines the outcome, and that's not really how the process has to be. We can make a conscious decision not to react. And when you make that discovery – and it really is like a discovery – it's like discovering a gold mine. When you make that discovery, you can, all of a sudden, not react to things that your children do, or things that your partner, your spouse, or coworker may do. Think of when someone has said something to you, even a total stranger, and it has set the tone for a whole day; it has, in the words of so many people, "ruined my day." You don't need to let anything or anybody "ruin" your day when you realize you have the ability not to take that downward spiral. You'll find yourself reacting to things throughout your day, but then saying, "Wait a second, I'm not going there. I'm just not going there." It cannot only give you a huge change in the way you live your life, or whether you have a good day or bad day, but I also think that it has an amazing impact on your stress level, and ultimately, on your health.

Gary: It has an impact on your health and on your ability to care for your loved ones.

Joan: Yes, and the ability to care for your loved one. When you start to understand what your partner, your children, or the other people in your own life are doing for their own reasons, it allows you to understand that they are reacting as well. Jonathan Cabbott Zen wrote the book *Wherever You Go, There You Are*, and the whole idea behind the book is that we see things through the glasses we choose to put on. It's just a wonderful concept because you realize that you can put a different set of glasses on. My mother always said to me when I was growing up, "Always have your rose colored glasses on." She was one of these "the glass is half full" people and the ultimate positive thinker, and some of it must have sunk in. However, it wasn't until later in life that I started my own kind of journey into meditation and into a different way of looking at things, and started reading about it, discovering authors like Jonathan Cabbott Zen, that I was finally saying, "Oh yeah, that's what my mother was talking about."

Gary: It really is important to caregivers to think like this because we're always looking for the next piece of bad news, or we're constantly placed in a reactionary mood.

Joan: The world that we live in these days makes you feel so overwhelmed with all the things you've got to keep up with, or catch up with, and all of a sudden to discover that you have the ability to make such a positive impact upon people's lives; that you actually have a lot more power than you think changes you, whether it's emotional (how you react to things), or whether it's your ability to impact them physically.

Gary: For example, you want to be sure that your kids establish a healthy lifestyle from the start...

Joan: Yes. I just spent the last year working with a pediatric nutritionist, Dr. Myron Winnick. He based his life-long studies and body of work on how we feed our children and how early nutrition will impact them when they are adults. If somebody said to you that they had an inoculation or a pill that you could give your child that would prevent them from getting any debilitating diseases such as adult diabetes, cancer, high blood pressure or coronary artery disease, and it would extend their lives by 10 to 15 years, you would say "Sign me up," and "Where do I get in line?" As parents, we actually do have that ability to impact our children's heath, but the problem is that so many people don't take their own health seriously; they don't exercise, don't eat right, and eat too much fast food and foods with transfats.

Gary: That's one reason why I like the American Heart Association's "Choose to Move" program. It is proactive, and it allows people to take whatever time they can during the day to care for themselves.

Joan: We know that women primarily make the decisions at the grocery store. They are the ones who cook the food and serve the meals. An organization like American Heart Association understands that you've got to focus on these women. You have to try to help them raise their awareness about cardiovascular disease, and how much we have in our own control. Thirty percent or so is due to our genetics and there's nothing you can really do about that, other than be aware of it; but 70 percent is within our control. How much more empowered do you want to be than that? You can have a significant impact on the outcome of your life, how long you live, and whether your years will be fun-filled and healthy.

Gary: How does this program work?

Joan: It's a free program and people can call 888-My-Heart or go to AmericanHeart.org/choosetomove. Choose to Move is really smart in taking a realistic approach, asking "What are people going to be able to put into their lives without having to make significant changes?" If you tell someone that they've got to join some huge exercise program, you're going to lose them. You're going to lose 75 percent of them within the first couple of weeks. They are just never going to do it. So the American Heart Association took the approach that they would find things that would be much more realistic for people to do. If we can just be their inspiration and they follow some of the suggestions about incorporating physical fitness, shopping wisely and eating more healthy foods, after only 12 weeks, I'm really convinced that they are going to feel better. Anyone who has said that they didn't have the energy to work out finds that after doing so, they have so much more energy. I think that when you come back from exercising, it gives you more patience, and makes you much more relaxed as a caregiver.

Gary: Have you been successful in communicating the message to caregivers who need the program?

Joan: Whenever I talk to a women's group, I tell them that if they make this investment in themselves, it will determine the quality of their lives five years from now or even 10 years from now. They will find that they'll be a better mom, a better partner, a better coworker and a better friend because they are going to be happier, more relaxed and have more energy. It's funny, but at 39-years-of-age, I was the woman I now preach to; I was 45 pounds overweight, never exercised and ate terribly. My wake-up call, ironically enough, was sitting on the set of *Good Morning America* and interviewing a representative of the American Heart Association. Their representative was giving our viewers a 10-question quiz as to their risk of cardiovascular disease. As I was listening to the questions, I realized that I had just flunked that test. It was like a light bulb going off in my head, and I really wanted to take this seriously. I didn't want to be watching the race, I wanted to be running in the race and thank God I did. Here I am now, in my 50s with two sets of twins under the age of two! I guarantee you that I am much healthier today than I was at 35. I know by making that commitment to myself, I've added years to my life and that I've made a huge impact on my family.

Gary: As caregivers, we tend to take ourselves out of the circle of care; making sure that our loved ones have everything they need, but ignoring our own needs. So it seems as if the road to becoming a better caregiver begins with taking better care of you.

Joan: It's just by nature that woman are caregivers, with everyone on these gigantic "to do" lists, your kids, your spouse, your boss—everybody but you. If you are able to cross 10 things off of the list, the item called "taking care of you," will end up being one of those things that will float to yet another list. The truth, is if we took better care of ourselves, then we'd be much more capable of attacking everything on our lists.

INTERVIEW WITH HECTOR ELIZONDO

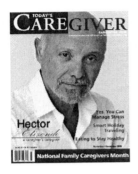

NOV / DEC 2008

Gary Barg: What were the first signs of your mother's Alzheimer's disease?

Hector Elizondo: The first signs of her illness were very subtle; just forgetfulness, the usual stuff, the shopping list, the keys, and then a pattern started to emerge. Realizing that now in retrospect, back then it was, "Oh Mom, please, you asked that question before, you know, a half hour ago." But the first real red flag was when she lost her way in her neighborhood.

Gary: They used to call Alzheimer's pre-senile dementia.

Hector: That's what she was diagnosed with. She was diagnosed with pre-senile dementia. We had no idea what the heck it meant; quite frankly, we had no idea what she had. No one had any idea about anything and my father, of course, was the primary caregiver. He's the one who took the brunt of the 24/7 care. You can imagine, especially in the Latino culture, you take care of your own; you don't go outside of it. And that's not uncommon for many other cultures except in the contiguous United States perhaps; you just took care of your own. There was no thought of doing it otherwise; but again, there was no thought of doing it otherwise because we had no other options. We had no information. There are many aspects of culture that make that up. My father would say, "This is something I've done. I'm being paid back."

Gary: He blamed himself.

Hector: Yes, of course, oh yes. "It must have been something I've done. Why is this happening?" And I always thought, living the life isn't enough? Isn't that hard enough? I mean, someone has to impose this punishment on you?

Gary: Where did he reach out? According to a Stanford University study a few years ago, 40 percent of Alzheimer's caregivers pass away before their loved ones do.

Hector: My father did. He had a nervous breakdown and his immune system went south, and that was it. Otherwise, a very healthy man all his life, but he smoked two packs a day; but back then, everybody did. He came from that generation. He reached out for help in the late stages when he started deteriorating physically to a point where he just couldn't do it anymore.

Gary: What would you suggest to family members now, when their loved ones are diagnosed with Alzheimer's, or they suspect Alzheimer's?

Hector: First of all, there's a possibility, or more than a possibility of being diagnosed. We really didn't get a real diagnosis. No one said this is what you have and this is what is going to happen; and it's a collective effort. You have to make these efforts as a family; try not to lose patience with Mom. She's going to ask the same question within five minutes. She may start losing her memory entirely. She may become incontinent. The list goes on and on. No one said that to us. So, that's why I feel so strongly about it.

Gary: I know you lived close to your parents at some point during this. Did your dad accept your help at all?

Hector: He accepted mine. He accepted help from the family, reluctantly. At one time, I even took my mother away. I was working and I said "Dad, I want to take her with me." It was a situation where I would have someone look after her. I made that arrangement. That didn't last and I said, "Okay, Dad, you go away, take a break of two weeks. Two weeks is good; that's it, don't worry about it. I can handle this." I was much younger, you know; I had the strength and resiliency to do that. It didn't go very well. He returned after a few days, maybe four or five days; that's it, he was back, couldn't take it. It was his responsibility and he was going to put a shoulder to the wheel; meanwhile, he was falling apart.

Gary: As you go around and people are learning about your family's story, are caregivers sharing their stories with you?

Hector: Oh yes, oh yes; it's a tsunami of information. It's a tsunami of sharing. They can hardly wait. Yes, of course. We were at a forum in San Francisco talking, the heads were nodding; they all had direct experiences with that. It's a terrible thing. But it doesn't have to be today. That's the wonderful thing. If my father had been around today, it would have been a different story.

Gary: That's one of the things we've noticed at our Fearless Caregiver Conferences over the last ten years; the best advice and support and the thing that opens their eyes is their time with their fellow caregivers.

Hector: Yes, they are involved with the community. They are not isolated. It's like being in AA. There are other people with it. You are not alone. When there is support, there's hope. It's as simple as that.

Gary: If you had one piece of advice that you would like to leave family and caregivers with, what would that be?

Hector: At the risk of sounding esoteric, we only have two real enemies in the world and that's ignorance and fear. That's it. The rest is ho-ha. There's no reason to be ignorant about the situation now. There is no reason to fear it. Get help. Simple.

GARY'S NOTE: PATRICIA RICHARDSON

Pat came in from New York to join us at the 2011 New Haven Fearless Caregiver Conference as her own home in Connecticut had lost power days earlier in the massive snow storm that hit the state so hard. We were grateful that the weather was absolutely perfect the day of the event. She and her puppy Olive left New York early to be with us for as much of the day as possible. Pat was a little concerned that we had her listed as keynote speaker since she really would rather interact with her fellow caregivers than give a speech. She had nothing to worry about. Once Pat stood up to speak, her conversation was personal and interactive— talking about her challenges as caregiver to a strong-willed dad, helping her sister through the sudden death of her brother-in-law, and the need to standardize the laws for "taking away drivers' licenses" when necessary.

What really impressed me was when she took all questions asked of her and shared advice with the family caregivers in the room. When Pat spoke of the guilt associated with the possibility of long-term care placement for her dad, a caregiver in the room responded with a story of her own feelings of guilt. This caregiver shared her own journey to the realization that it would be better for her entire family for her own dad to live in an appropriate long-term care facility. As national spokesperson for CUREPSP, an organization for those living with the disease that claimed her dad's life, Pat is a care advocate. But at the event, she was simply one of the caregivers who were sharing stories and learning from one another. In fact, as a caregiver said of the day, "Hey, this is like a big support group!" Exactly right.

INTERVIEW WITH PATRICIA RICHARDSON

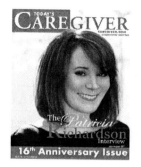

JUL / AUG 2011

Gary Barg: I appreciate you talking about your dad. I think when we talk about our families, and especially people in the public eye like yourself, it really makes a difference and brings people out who may be going through this. It is a great service that you do. Could you tell us what PSP is?

Patricia Richardson: Progressive supranuclear palsy (PSP) is a neurodegenerative brain disease that has no known cause, treatment or cure. It affects nerve cells that control walking, balance, mobility, vision, speech and swallowing. We used to say movement disorder, but we have decided now to refer to it as a disease. That's what it is and when you say a movement disorder, it does not sound as serious and deadly as it in fact is. It is a fatal disease. It is a fatal brain disease.

We did not even know my father had it, probably for the first five years. Towards the last probably full year he had it, and maybe even longer, I used to say to people that it was like he was mummified inside his body. He had the kind of PSP where the muscle cramps basically froze him. He was unable to move his face or eyes. Of course, he could not speak for more than the last year, probably the last two years, and he had a lot of difficulty swallowing.

We had never known how cognitive he had actually been because he could not communicate. Then when we did the autopsy, we found out that he had been a lot more aware than we realized. That was so upsetting to us, because there were times when we talked in front of him and did not think he necessarily really even understood what we were saying. Now we realize he did; he understood a lot more about what was going on around him than we realized at the time.

Gary: That is a good lesson for everybody with a loved one dealing with cognitive disorders or movement disorders. We should try to be aware of what the person may or may not be processing. What kinds of treatments are being developed for PSP? What was being done for your dad?

Patricia: When my father died six years ago, there was not anything even close to treat PSP. There are several different strains of PSP, and he had the strain of PSP that was the Parkinsonian type. That was just one of the things that confused us further because when he was diagnosed wrongly with Parkinson's, it seemed that he was initially responding to the medication. People who have the Parkinsonian type can sometimes respond to Parkinsonian meds, at least initially, and he did for a while. One thing I want to be sure and mention is there is a kind of treatment called VitalStim Therapy that can help with speaking or swallowing. The treatment is done by a speech therapist. They put these electrodes on their throat and have them try to speak or swallow at the same time. It got my father speaking again for another couple of months and he could speak while he was doing the therapy; and it kept him swallowing until he died. This therapy was miraculous. I am convinced if it had not worked out, my father would have had to use a feeding tube.

Gary: You were also a long-distance caregiver for both your parents?

Patricia: My parents both took 10 years to die, give or take. My mother had so many different diseases and then had a stroke; it was one thing after another. It was a long, slow, steady decline and loss before my mother finally left. Neither one of them were themselves one day and the next day died. This was not the way they expected to go. It was so shocking and so horrible. My sisters and I went through a long process where we would take turns visiting them. My parents insisted on retiring where none of us lived because they did not want to be a burden for us. It ended up being so much more difficult because it meant that every time there was a health crisis, of which there were many, we would have to take turns going there. So it would be me first because being a celebrity helps get attention at the hospital. Then we would go in tandem, one after another, so that there would be somebody there longer.

Gary: It is what we call the professionalization of family caregiving.

Patricia: Also, I really do not trust nursing homes. We had the best nursing home in Virginia Beach and my dad got hurt by a nurse there. They covered it up. They did not file an accident report. They hid it. They did not put it in the records. They did not even tell his doctor. Only because I happened to turn up and I had a caregiver in the room with him every day did we find out. One of the things I learned, and that I would tell the caregivers, is if you have a family member in a nursing home, never visit the same time of day. Go and show up at

6:00 in the morning. Show up at 8:00 at night. Never let them know when you are coming. You have to stay on top of them.

Gary: That is exactly right.

Patricia: And make sure you are checking all over their bodies to be sure they do not have sores. If there is an incident ever, if you see that there is some kind of infection going on or something that happened, you check their chart to be sure it was marked there. Make sure that there was an incident report. These facilities are supposed to be reporting if there is any kind of incident. If it is not in there, you raise Cain. I just had to learn these lessons the hard way. There were really horrible things that happened and we learned the hard way.

Gary: The result is that you raised the visibility of your dad from being the patient in room 201 to being someone that people are really looking in on and caring about.

Patricia: Yes, but you have to be careful. We found out that some of the nurses were calling my father King Larry because they resented that. On the other hand, we heard there were people that had families who lived in town and did not have visits like my dad got. Even though they may have resented him and called him King Larry, I do not think they dared do anything to him after that. They were worried because they knew we were watching.

Gary: That is right. I think that is worth its weight in gold.

Patricia: Yes, that is the thing. Most of the nurses really mean well. You want to have a good relationship with them and treat them with the respect they deserve, but it is like a two-handed thing. On the one hand, you want to treat them with respect and have a good relationship. On the other hand, do not count on anything.

Gary: You mean you should trust, but verify, and it is a partnership. You cannot immediately assume everyone is going to be terrible, but you cannot immediately assume that you are going to get the best care the system has to offer.

Patricia: Your parent cannot tell you. They have no way to tell you what is really happening. Sometimes your loved one will try to communicate to you. Sometimes you will sense that they are hearing something or that they are uncomfortable with someone. If you get that feeling, trust it and try to figure out a way to get your loved one to communicate to you.

Get a white board. See if they can scratch something out on the white board. I did that with Dad for a while. What was hilarious was when I finally got that idea and got a white board and magic marker for him to scrawl something out, it was really hard to read. What was the first thing he wrote after months of not being able to communicate to us? You would think it would be I love you or blah, blah, blah. Guess what he wrote?

Gary: Go ahead.

Patricia: Vanilla milkshake, vanilla milkshake, vanilla milkshake. That is what we got. Vanilla milkshake. I was like, okay, you got it. I was off to get one.

Gary: Can you tell me a little bit more about CurePSP?

Patricia: The Web site is CurePSP.org. Now we are helping people with CBD (corticobasal degeneration). We are helping people with MSA (multiple system atrophy) and a couple other rare brain diseases. We are covering more than just PSP. CBD is close to PSP in so many of the symptoms. We are helping people with CBD and also doing research as much as we are in PSP. We are helping the caregivers with MSA. Then we are helping a couple of the other rare diseases that just would not be able to have an organization of their own. That is why we changed our name to CurePSP: Foundation for PSP, CBD and Related Brain Diseases.

Gary: What would be the one piece of information you would really love to leave them with as a family caregiver?

Patricia: When we were going through this with my dad, we did not have the help of CurePSP. We did not even know about the Web site. I really believe that the most important thing is to get with a group. Go online, find out everything you can about the disease and find other people like you who are going through what you are going through. They are going to be with you. Your loved ones are going to see other people like themselves. If you go to meetings, not only are you going to be with other caregivers that you can share what you are going through with, but your loved one is going to see other people going through what they are going through.

INTERVIEW WITH BRUCE JENNER

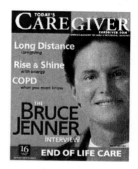

MAR / APR 2011

Gary Barg: Can you tell me about the DRIVE4COPD program and how your trip went?

Bruce Jenner: First of all, why did I do it? The reason I did it is because both my wife's grandparents died of emphysema. When you talk about caregiving, the rest of the family becomes the caregiver to people who are afflicted by this and it is just such a strain on everybody; not just the patient, but also the caregiver. COPD is the fourth leading killer in the United States. So that is the reason we did it; to build awareness of what COPD is. Why do we want them to be aware? Because there are a lot of things you can do to help manage this disease along the way, to make the quality of life better. Now they say there are approximately 24 million people affected by COPD. Half of them don't know they even have the problem.

As we went across the United States, it was kind of the race for the missing millions, those twelve million people who are affected by this who do not know they even have the disease. They just think, "I am getting a little old, a little winded or I got this little cough." Early detection is extremely important. We are trying to make people aware and drive them to the Web site, which is DRIVE4COPD.com, and also take the screener to see if you are at risk. It has been very successful.

Gary: What should I be looking for to be worried about myself or a loved one having COPD?

Bruce: Coughing, chronic coughing, coughing up a lot of mucous, shortness of breath when you do normal daily activities where a few years ago, you would not even notice your breathing. Now all of a sudden, you notice that you are breathing hard. You walk up the stairs and you are having a hard time getting your breath.

Obviously, you are at risk if you smoke or have been smoking for a long period of time, or maybe have the disease in your family. It also depends on what type of working conditions you have, how good the air quality has been throughout your life, things like that. You just have to be aware, because most people do not realize they have it until the latter stages and then it is harder to manage.

Gary: What kind of reaction have you had from people on the road?

Bruce: I had people with oxygen masks come up and stand in line saying thank you for building up the awareness for this. What I was also trying to do is encourage young people who are really not at risk to listen to their parents and if they are coughing away, to put the test in front of them. See how they score and, depending on how they score, maybe go see a specialist and get checked out. So, even young people who are not at risk as much can really do something about this, too.

Gary: It seems like you got a lot of appreciation for what you have been doing.

Bruce: Yes. The response has been just phenomenally good. You know, COPD is the fourth leading cause of death in the United States. One person every four minutes dies of COPD. It is the only disease that is on the rise because, for example, we can do things for treating breast cancer and we have gotten better at managing diabetes. Yet, too many people find out they have emphysema so late in the process and they have lost so much function, there is not much we can do about it. So COPD is on the rise.

Gary: So that has to be hard for you. I mean, being a world class Olympian, to see people around you who you love and who cannot breathe.

Bruce: It is the worst thing in the world. You cannot even imagine. When you watch them, it is almost like they are drowning. They just cannot get the air in.

Gary: I was wondering if you and Kris have had conversations with your adult children about your advanced directive wishes.

Bruce: Kris and I have discussed that, but not too much with the kids. We put it in the will how we wanted to be treated. To be honest with you, we just, in the last month, had to deal with that with a very close friend. She was here for Christmas and three days later went into a coma and was basically in a vegetative state, but was technically still alive. Our kids are very close to her children. They all grew up together and we all dealt with this together. Eventually, it was the consensus of her family (the two sons and this woman's brother) to turn the machines off when there was no chance that it was going to work out for her. So, yes, these are tough decisions that every family, or pretty much every family, has to deal with at some point. At what point is there quality of life or not? I am more of a quality of life man. If I am that bad off that you are even thinking about this, yes, let me go in peace.

Gary: If you had one takeaway piece of advice for a family caregiver, what would your one most important piece of advice be for them?

Bruce: We have a very large blended family, a lot of dynamics. The most important thing you can do as parents is to work hard to keep a good strong family bond. If somebody gets in trouble, we can rally behind them. If somebody gets sick, we are going to rally behind them. They always know that their family will be there for them. I think that is probably the most important thing; to have a strong family bond and do everything you can to keep that bond strong.

▪◼ **GARY'S NOTE:** HENRY WINKLER

I'm sure that I am talking out of school, but the overriding comments I heard from all of the public relations and advocacy folks I spoke with when arranging the interview with Henry Winkler and his appearance at the Western Connecticut Fearless Caregiver Conference was that he is, by far, the nicest person in Hollywood. Frankly, nothing that I heard from him at the event disproved that contention. In fact, he spoke with the audience for over an hour and then took as many questions as there were hands raised. He would always ask the questioner to say their name before they launched into their question. One attendee stood up and as I brought the microphone over to her I saw that she was, quite frankly, shaking. She said her name was Amy and that she grew up with the Fonz's pictures plastered across her bedroom. As a teenager, Amy bought every magazine he was in and never missed an episode of *Happy Days* when the show was on the air. She told Henry that this was a moment she had been dreaming about for nearly 40 years. Without skipping beat, Henry responded, "I've been waiting all this time to meet you, too, Amy." The nicest guy in Hollywood and at that moment, in Southbury, Connecticut, as well.

INTERVIEW WITH HENRY WINKLER

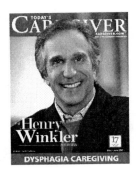

MAY / JUN 2012

Gary Barg: Let me start by saying, Welcome, Mr. Ambassador.

Henry Winkler: Thank you.

Gary: I know that you have an OBE Knighthood from the Queen of England, but you are also the Ambassador for the Open Arms Campaign to help educate people about upper limb spasticity [ULS]. How did you get involved in the campaign?

Henry: Well, my mother had a stroke in '89 causing upper limb spasticity. I saw what happened to her, and then I saw what happens when you have a brand new tool to help possibly alleviate the upper limb spasticity. From listening to all the doctors I've toured with, I've learned that upper limb spasticity often develops about three or four months after a stroke when the patient is home. The regular visits are over; maybe even the physical therapy, and the secondary muscles of the arms compensate, take over and seize up. And you've seen it a million times. You've seen a hand that is crumpled. An arm that is twisted and frozen against the body. A palm that is closed and the fingernails are growing into the palm. And that is a generalized view of upper limb spasticity. It works on the ego because it's unsightly. People judge the body because the body is different.

Gary Barg: Right.

Henry: I've seen the results of this therapeutic use of Botox with my own eyes and it's pretty incredible to me. It is a pleasure to go around and talk about this and just bring the information to caregivers, doctors and patients and let them decide together if it is right for them. You don't get the use of your arm back—that is a whole other therapy if it comes back; but it's easier to live with. It's less painful. It is easier for the caregiver to help you get dressed. Without the therapy, people would have to buy a shirt, a dress or a t-shirt three to four sizes too big for the person just to get their arm through.

Gary: And honestly, it's an emotional help, too, if you can imagine.

Henry: You know what? That is exactly correct. That, I think, is a major, major component—the emotional.

Gary: They don't feel so helpless.

Henry: You don't feel so helpless, you don't feel so freakish, you don't feel so different. There was a woman I met in Texas who had her arm frozen to the side of her body and she called it her chicken wing. Her children who had given up their social life to take care of her called it her chicken wing. And you know, when she started the therapeutic use of Botox, she said, "I haven't been able to put my arms around my girls for two years since the stroke. It's amazing... it's amazing." And you know what happens also that I'm privy to, that I am honored by? People in the get-togethers that we have had all over the country stand up and give testimony about where they were and what has happened. And it's almost, I don't want to say religious, but it is. It's like a revival.

Gary: It's sharing.

Henry: It's sharing, but it's sharing this monumental change that they so appreciate. I've never actually said that sentence, but that is the truth.

Gary: They bring something to the table that has helped them and again, giving is getting. The other thing that I love so much about the Open Arms Campaign is that it allows the care recipient to partner with their family caregiver.

Henry: That is a very good way to say it. All of a sudden, they become a part of the team as opposed to the object.

Gary: It is often so difficult for a parent to see your kids caring for you.

Henry: What about the parent caring for the kid? I just met a young man who was on his way to becoming a doctor like his dad. His sisters are 14 and 15. They were on vacation when he was 18 or 19 and he had a stroke. He is working his way, fighting his way back.

Gary: And he is affected by ULS?

Henry: Yes.

Gary: Aren't people living with MS and some other diseases also affected by ULS?

Henry: There are so many—head injury, cerebral palsy, stroke, of course, spinal cord injury.

Gary: By the way, the stories on the campaign's Web site, openarmscampaign.com, are the kind of stories we hear all the time through the Fearless Caregiver Conferences and *Today's Caregiver* magazine, but the pictures of the family members are amazing. You just see people getting part of their life back. Do you meet a lot of family caregivers on the road?

Henry: I do, indeed.

Gary: What kind of stories do they tell you?

Henry: They tell me that it really, really helped them. It helped them be a better caregiver. It helped their job. It helped their patient. It helped their parent. It helped their child. They are just grateful.

Gary: How many folks in the country are going through this?

Henry: Over a million. A million people have had a stroke in America and a tremendous amount of those get upper limb spasticity.

Gary: That's amazing. What were people doing before?

Henry: Living with it. Struggling with it.

Gary: What is the one most important piece of advice you have for family caregivers?

Henry: I'd say I have two things. One is make sure that your glass is half full so you can present that glass to the people you work with. That's number one. I think everything comes from self-image. I really do.

Gary: That's excellent. And your second one?

Henry: And my second one is tenacity. That somehow you keep the fire burning to take those tiny steps forward because it is so easy to just give up.

Gary: Absolutely. And so, then, the number one thing you have to do is care for yourself first.

Henry: Yeah, that's right. That's in everything. I so agree with that. I always say that if you don't get it together with your own personal self, you can't do much.

Gary: You can be no help to anyone else.

Henry: That's right. Believe it or not, when I speak publicly—not about this, necessarily, just when I'm speaking, I end my speech with that very thought. You know, there is no altruism, actually. That's a concept that is, I think, unlivable. You do something nice and it feels good. You are also doing it for yourself.

Gary: Right. You can't ignore yourself.

Henry: You can't ignore yourself. There is nothing wrong with not ignoring yourself as long as your circle widens to include at least one other human being.

INTERVIEW WITH PHYLICIA RASHAD

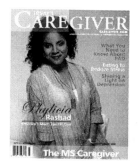

JAN / FEB 2009

Gary Barg: What should people know about PAD [peripheral artery disease]?

Phylicia Rashad: That the people who are at greatest risk for developing PAD are those with diabetes who are over 50 years old, who have hypertension, high cholesterol, people who are heavy smokers, people over 70; people with a history of heart attack or a stroke in their family.

Gary: How has PAD affected your family?

Phylicia: When I did hear about PAD, I thought about my father immediately, because my father had diabetes and he died of a heart attack. Then I continued to read about PAD and I remember the moment that I read about one of the common symptoms, and that is the cramping in the legs. The first thing that struck me was those risk factors. So, when I read about that, I really thought about my dad then because he used to complain about that. His legs would cramp and we thought it was because he had been practicing dentistry for almost 35 years, standing up the whole time because he refused to sit down. You could attribute it to that. Oftentimes when people have discomfort in their legs, it is attributed to being tired, or they think, "I have been standing too long; oh, I am getting older." Not considering that there could be a cardiovascular problem at the root of this.

Gary: It sounds like it makes a lot of sense to educate yourself about the risk factors and then be in honest communication with your loved ones to determine if they are at risk.

Phylicia: If you have these risk factors, or if you just want to know, you can ask for the A.B.I. test. That is the Ankle-Brachial Index test which involves taking the blood pressure at both arms and then at both ankles. The diagnosis for PAD is significant in that PAD is a warning there is poor circulation in your arteries in your legs. If there is poor circulation in your arteries and your legs, there is poor circulation in arteries leading to the heart and to the brain.

Gary: So as in all things, knowledge in this case is power.

Phylicia: Knowledge is power.

Gary: What is a PAD hotspot?

Phylicia: A PAD hotspot is an area in which there is a prevalence of PAD diagnosis, or people who are at risk.

Gary: Are there things that you and your loved one can do to help prevent PAD, like diet and exercise? Are there risk factors that you might want to tell people they need to think about?

Phylicia: Absolutely; there are things I think about. There is a family history. In my family, there is a medical history of diabetes on both parents' sides. My mother's father had diabetes. He died of a stroke. My father, his parents, and his siblings all had diabetes. If you know that it is there, then you need to pay attention to the way you are living. You should pay attention to the way you are living anyway, but given that family medical history, you know there is stuff you need to do.

You need to exercise. You need to pay very close attention to your diet. I have to do that. It is not a problem for me because I enjoy healthy foods. But I take it even a step further. I have gone so far as to find out about food sensitivities, because all healthy foods do not go well with this body. I was not always aware of that, but I am aware of it now. I pay close attention to nutrition and things I do to supplement my nutrition.

Gary: As you travel the country, have you gotten a response from people living with PAD?

Phylicia: Within recent months, a friend of mine, who smoked heavily for many years, called me to say—this was her exact wording—she said, "Hey, I'm maxed out; they want to take my leg." She had had a problem with her toe. She had injured it somehow and it wasn't healing properly. We had been speaking on and off prior to this and it was not getting better. She said they tell me I have PAD and I have developed gangrene. Because of my work with the PAD Coalition, I was able to put her in contact with one of those chief physicians in the Coalition who directed her to a physician in her home town who was able to spare her leg. She lost some toes, but she was able to keep her leg. But you see, that is the thing—she never even put it together that her smoking was the root cause of her problem. It was not the injury that she sustained. It was the fact that she had been smoking for so long that it had affected her circulation.

Then after all of this is said and done, then she says, "Well yes, my leg did start feeling kind of cold, I would notice that my leg felt cold." Well, yes, it felt cold because there was no circulation there. People do not put these things together.

Gary: I think that story is an inspiration for others in her kind of situation. It is the sharing and the communicating that make the difference and not being afraid of picking up the phone; and if you do not get the right support from your physician, move on.

If you only had one piece of advice for somebody about their own healthcare or about caring for their loved one, what would that advice be?

Phylicia: You must take care of yourself. It is an act of love. You should take care of yourself so that you are really nurturing yourself to have the best to give to others. From my own experience, it is important to take care of one's own self. Not as self defense, not as an act of revenge or rage, but because it is the right thing to do.

If there is no water in the well, you cannot share it with people. If there is no food in the refrigerator, you cannot feed people. If there is no energy in your body, if your mind is in a state of constant distraction or dismay, you cannot be of service to people. And you are not going to be the best company either.

GARY'S NOTE: LINDA DANO

We were joined by our friend Linda Dano and her friend, Mo, a beautiful 10-year-old Lhasa Apso, at our New Haven Fearless Caregiver Conference in 2007. Linda brought the message of the importance of having support partners as you care. She believes so much in the value of support in beating depression that she has been going around the country talking to caregivers about the concept. Linda, who had been dealing with an emotional whirlwind over the past few years, was a caregiver for her father who was living with Alzheimer's. Soon after her father passed a few years ago, her loving husband and mother passed away within days of each other. She was devastated; and just as she started to find her bearings once again, she lost her beloved dog Charlie. But Linda was not there necessarily to talk about her struggles, but her recovery. What the audience gleaned from Linda's heartfelt message was that no matter what you are living through, there is hope. One other small thing—my brother Steven will never forget that event since he (for the first time ever) had to go on stage and stall while Linda and I spent an additional ten minutes talking about our dogs.

INTERVIEW WITH LINDA DANO

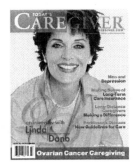

SEPT / OCT 2006

Gary Barg: How did you become a caregiver?

Linda Dano: I'm originally from California; when I moved to New York 22 years ago, my mother and father remained in California. In the early 1990s, my mother began telling me that my dad was forgetting things and acting differently. Eventually, it got to the point where it was becoming exceedingly difficult for my mother to handle my father, but we still had no idea it was Alzheimer's disease. My dad was "cranky," his increasing forgetfulness would make him really angry — angry in a way that wasn't like him. So, my husband Frank and I both decided to ask my parents if they could come to New York and live with us.

Gary: When were you told that the diagnosis was Alzheimer's disease?

Linda: On Thanksgiving morning my father fell. We thought he had broken his hip because he was screaming in pain. At this point he wasn't talking, he was only babbling and yelling — he was completely out of control. After the fall, we got him admitted to Mt. Sinai Hospital. But because his hip wasn't broken and he was still very agitated, the only place they could put him was the psychiatric ward. Still, no one, not one doctor, suggested that my dad might have Alzheimer's.

My dad hated the psych ward. After being admitted, he stopped eating and I was told that I should give him a feeding tube. I did because I didn't know what else to do. They told me that we couldn't possibly keep him at home; he was too strong and he was becoming increasingly violent. At this point, I met Dr. Robert Butler, who was head of Geriatrics at Mt. Sinai. Dr. Butler was at the forefront of Alzheimer's disease research and treatment. It was Dr. Butler who got my dad out of the psych ward and helped me admit him to an appropriate nursing home in New York City...something I swore I would never do.

Gary: You must have been devastated. How did all this affect you?

Linda: At first I really went in blinded because I didn't want to believe it. How could my father have Alzheimer's? Then, when the diagnosis did come, I was relieved to know that there was a reason for my dad's behavior, and that he wasn't crazy. It was the most traumatic experience of my entire life, watching my dad every day get further and further and further away from us.

Gary: What were the things that provided your greatest support back then?

Linda: My husband's support and the fact that I was able to save my mother in the process. Had my mother dealt with my father alone away from me, I'm not sure she would have survived. I think it would have taken her down along with my dad. By bringing my mother to be with me in New York,

I truly believe that I saved her. I'm so thankful for that.

Gary: What suggestions do you have for people getting into the same situation?

Linda: I believe that people must have a third ear and a third eye when looking at their loved ones — you need to look for warning signs. If you have elderly parents and grandparents, you need to REALLY look at them; don't write off changes in behavior or memory as a normal part of aging. If they're starting to behave differently, you need to have them checked out to see why. You need a proper diagnosis because until you do, you don't know what you're dealing with and you can't put together a plan. You don't over-react. You don't react in a hysterical way, which is what I did. You know what to do.

Gary: It seems like one of the biggest challenges for an Alzheimer's caregiver is watching a loved one's mind just slipping away. It's not like cancer or anything else where the mind is...

Linda: Is still there. You keep hoping there's some little glint in their eye that they know you. One Sunday night, I came in from Connecticut to the nursing home and my father was in bed. It was about 10:00 at night and I patted his face and I said, "Hi, Poppa," and he opened his eyes and he said, "Hi, Linda." It was all that I could do not to get him dressed and take him home. It was the only time he ever said my name where I really believed he knew it was me...just for an instant, and then, it went away again. I cried over that for days.

Gary: Once you accept the fact that the person is gone from you and something happens and they're able to come back for a few seconds, it's really a tough...

Linda: It's like a rollercoaster ride.

Gary: That's a perfect way to put it. Did you go to a support group?

Linda: No. I didn't do any of it. I just lived with my own pain and I didn't talk about it to anybody. I wasn't making good decisions. I was so guilt-ridden that I didn't go and get information. What was the point? My father had already left me — that was my thinking. I couldn't save him now. I just ate and beat myself up and cried. I never, ever went to the nursing home that I didn't sit on the back staircase and weep before I'd go home.

Gary: What are the lessons learned?

Linda: We can't let feelings of guilt overtake us. We have to give ourselves a break. As a caregiver, you have to also take care of you. You have to reach out for help and you have to ask for help from anyone you can. You need to get into a support group. You need to share. You can't lose you in the process; you just can't. How can you really take care of someone else if you don't take care of yourself? You can't be strong for somebody else if you're a mess.

Gary: If you had only one piece of advice to share with a family caregiver, what would that be?

Linda: The common thread with caregivers is the emotional ride they all take: the isolation, feeling trapped, and then guilty that they feel that way. If I could say one thing to caregivers, it would be that they must reach out for help; they must! They have to ask for help from family and friends, whether that be a simple, "Please, can you set the table because I've got to go into the bathroom, and I've got to put myself in a tub for 10 minutes," or "I need to walk around the block. I need to get out. I need a break." Asking other family members to do things for the loved one, not taking it all on yourself. Also talking is very important. They must talk; share their feelings, their emotions, their fears and their anger. They must talk.

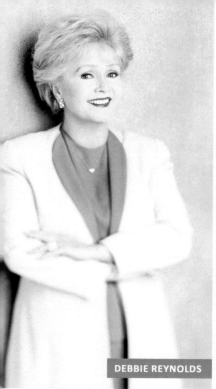

DEBBIE REYNOLDS

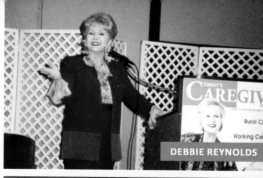

DEBBIE REYNOLDS

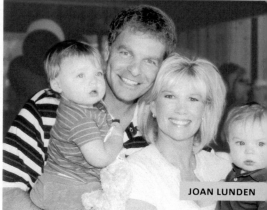

JOAN LUNDEN

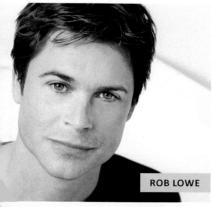

ROB LOWE

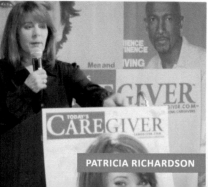

PATRICIA RICHARDSON

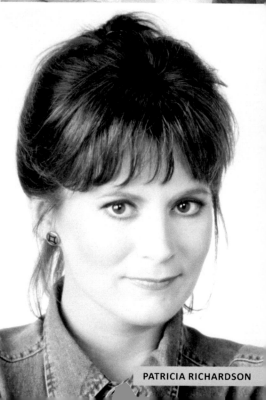

PATRICIA RICHARDSON

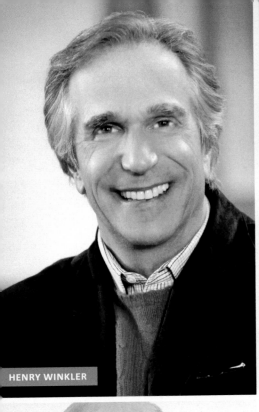

HENRY WINKLER

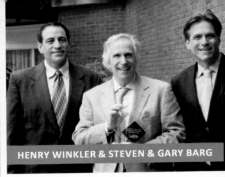

HENRY WINKLER & STEVEN & GARY BARG

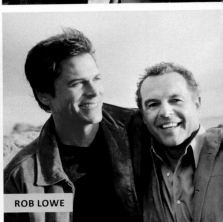

ROB LOWE

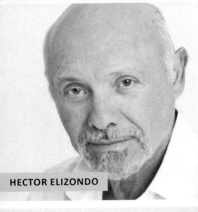

HECTOR ELIZONDO

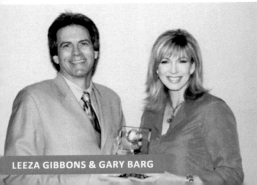

LEEZA GIBBONS & GARY BARG

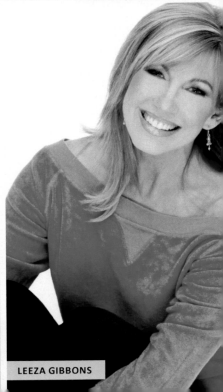

LEEZA GIBBONS

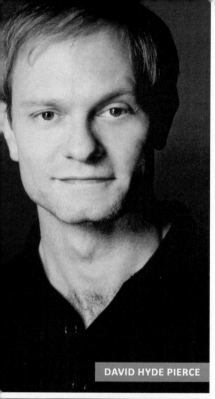

DAVID HYDE PIERCE

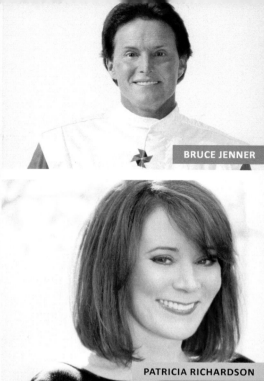

BRUCE JENNER

PATRICIA RICHARDSON

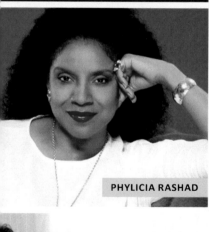

PHYLICIA RASHAD

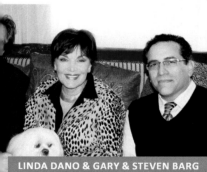

LINDA DANO & GARY & STEVEN BARG

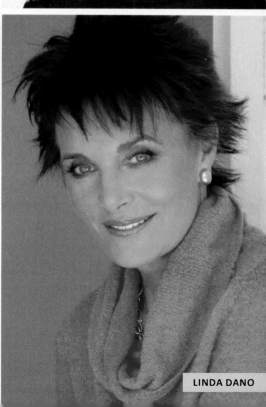

LINDA DANO

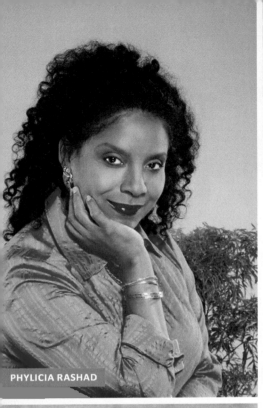

PHYLICIA RASHAD

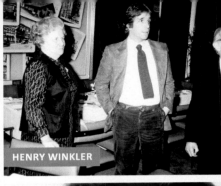

HENRY WINKLER

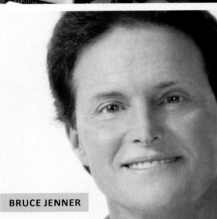

BRUCE JENNER

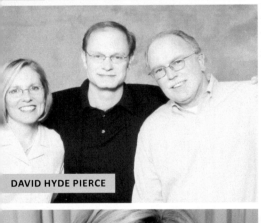

DAVID HYDE PIERCE

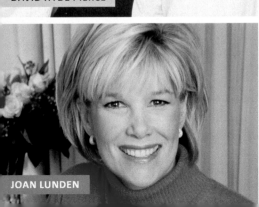

JOAN LUNDEN

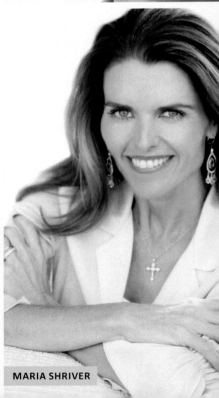

MARIA SHRIVER

Caring for PARTNERS

From my own experience, it is important to take care of one's own self. Not as self-defense, not as an act of revenge or rage, but because it is the right thing to do.

— Phylicia Rashad

GARY'S NOTE: GAIL SHEEHY

I knew that caregiving was about to hit the media map as a true life passage, as opposed to being seen as something that just happens to us, when Gail Sheehy wrote a book about it. Her 1970's breakthrough book *Passages* details the stages we go through during the years between 18 and 50, and her book *Passages in Caregiving* does the same for caregivers as we face the challenges of caring for our loved ones. I was very honored that our Fearless Caregiver work is mentioned in her book.

There was so very much to talk with Gail about and the interview went on for longer than usual. I was wondering how we could possibly cut it down to fit the allotted space in the magazine. It turns out I didn't have to worry. When I first saw Gail at a national conference, after she had received the copy of the issue in which she was interviewed, she gave our editor, Nancy Schonwalter, the best compliment possible when she said she thought the piece was extremely well edited. A well-deserved compliment from someone who knows her stuff.

INTERVIEW WITH GAIL SHEEHY

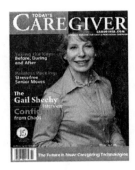

MAR / APR 2010

Gary Barg: So often, we find that it is a phone call in the middle of the night that marks the beginning of becoming a family caregiver. I was taken by the fact that your caregiving actually did start with a phone call.

Gail Sheehy: Yes. I think it usually does start with a call. Even with a creeping crisis, where nobody really wants to acknowledge that Mom is forgetting more than usual and sometimes cannot find her way home. It may go on for a year or two before there finally will be a crisis and Mom will be lost; or you will get a call because Dad has run a red light and he does not remember how he got into that accident.

My call was from my husband's surgeon, who two years before, had removed a cyst on Clay's neck, had it surveyed and it came back that it was benign. Then, these years later, I get a call saying, "You know the cyst on your husband's neck? We had the slides re-cut and it is actually cancer."

Suddenly, your world turns upside down. You are not just going to a concert that night; instead, you are thinking about how to save your husband's life. And he, like many men, approached it as just another job. So, we set out that way. How do we find the doctors? How do we evaluate one doctor from another?

Gary: You mentioned in the book that we need to find a medical quarterback and I thought that is great. Could you go into that a little bit?

Gail: Yes. We have so many specialists today, and they can be quite wonderful. But when you are dealing with a sudden, life threatening diagnosis, and you seek a second or even a third opinion, you have no idea how to compare all of these different perspectives. We do not know the lingo; we do not know what to do first. What I learned was that the most important thing is to find a doctor you trust who seems to have the largest perspective. Then ask that doctor if he or she will be your medical quarterback; take in the recommendations from everybody else and present you with a checklist of what you need to do.

Gary: One other thing I find very exciting about this kind of partnering with your loved one's care team is that it makes your loved one stand out.

Gail: I think it is amazing that you are saying we want to be part of the team. I think a huge part of successful treatment is feeling that the caregiver, patient, and health professional are working together. We will help, we will do research, we will work with you, but we want you to work with us as a collaborative team.

Gary: I really like your use of the phrase "labyrinth of caregiving" in the book. I think it is a very illuminating way to describe the caregiving experience. Please walk me through that concept.

Gail: Like everyone else, I felt like I was just in chaos; there was no structure to what we were going through. And then I was on a caregiver retreat in a church and I began walking a labyrinth that was inscribed on the floor. It felt very relaxing, serene and secure because you are walking a path that is laid out for you; then suddenly, there is a twist and you are going in reverse. You go along for a little while and then there is another twist, another sharp turn. I thought, wow, this is just like what I am going through as a caregiver.

As I proceeded, I saw that you have to have faith and you have to have patience, but this is a path. There is a way into it and there is a way out of it, if you just stay on the path and have faith. When I got to the center with a great sense of relief, I began to think that this must be the place where you know that your loved one is going to come back, or is going to become more and more needy and eventually leave you.

I came to understand that is the point at which you, the caregiver, have to begin preparing your own way back. You are on a different path than they are. Your mom, your dad, or maybe your spouse is on a path that ends with their leaving this world. You are on a path that has to bring you back into the world. That is a dual path and it is quite hard to think about, but it is nothing to feel guilty about. The greatest tragedy is if you lose two for one; when the caregiver goes down with the person they are caring for, and that happens much too often.

So, as I thought about it over the years that I was caregiving, I began to see that there were certain crisis points along the way that were quite commonplace. I came up with eight of them, or "Turnings." They are not linear, and you come back to ones that you have been over before; but you know them differently because you have been there and you know how to handle them.

The first Turning is Shock and Mobilization. That is when the call comes in. It is out of the blue, you are not prepared, and your life seems to be turned upside down; but often you do not really see yourself as a caregiver. You are just trying to get through the day. Your mobilization is in speaking with the doctors, dealing with the treatments and the conflicting opinions you will hear from family members. Ultimately, you and the person you are caring for have to retreat and process all that you have learned, come to a decision yourselves, and then go from there.

When the immediate crisis is over, you settle into the second Turning—A New Normal. It just happens naturally. In time, you gradually get accustomed to the new normal and you know that you can deal with it. This may go on for months, years, or even many years.

But, then there is the third stage—Boomerang. Almost inevitably, there will be another crisis of some sort. This time, you know it better and you are a little smarter about how to galvanize and mobilize. It is very important at this point to have a family meeting. If you let other members of the family go on just depending on you as the primary caregiver, you are going to burn out. It is very important to arrange the family meeting in such a way that you are not the boss; that you have a neutral and professional intermediary so everybody can feel as though they have important contributions to make.

Gary: Right, and this is where you learn to be the coach; to be able to say, "Okay, I have been here before; now I know what my informal network has to be." You pretty much know how to manage to the point where you have gotten yourself to the next step in the caregiving phase.

Gail: You, the primary caregiver, now need to graduate to care manager. Right? And you need to get used to thinking of yourself as a professional and presenting yourself that way to other health care professionals.

Gary: Absolutely.

Gail: The fourth Turning is called Playing God, which is when people who perform the caregiving role almost in isolation begin to think (I did, too) that you and you alone are responsible for keeping this person alive. The person you are taking care of will often reinforce that by saying things such things as, "My daughter is the only one I really trust," and this becomes a co-dependent relationship. The problem is that as long as things are going well and you are succeeding, your ego is stimulated by the idea of how important, how absolutely essential you are; you are playing God. And then, when something does not go well or the treatment backfires and you cannot catch up, well, if you are God, it is your fault. So, it is a no-win situation. Finally you have to get to the point where you say, if you are a believer, "There is a God, but I am not It."

Gary: But I will certainly be happy to partner with Him or Her.

Gail: Yes, but I will be a partner; exactly. And you know, ask for help every day. Say, "You know, dear God, there is nothing that can be thrown our way today that we cannot deal with together." As caregiver, it is not all on you.

The next Turning is I Can't Do This Anymore. Just saying those words is a signal that you have to call for help. You have to drop out once a day for at least an hour. You may only go out for 20 minutes the first time and just walk around the block. But when you realize that your loved one did not die in those 20 minutes, maybe you can do 40 minutes the next day. You work up to an hour, and that hour has to be nothing to do with caregiving; it's no fair calling the doctor about a prescription.

Then there is the Circle of Care; you will need to create a circle of people who will assume some responsibility for aspects of care. Let members of your family and friends who have not been involved know that you have reached the end of your rope. The Seventh Turning is called Coming Back. I think this may be the most important Turning of all. You know that your loved one might get well and stay well; but if you are still on this journey, you get to a point where you have to acknowledge that your loved one is not going to get well and is going to become more dependent. That is the point where you, as hard as it may sound, need to begin the letting go process. People who are able to begin that thought process begin preparing their own way back; you are on a different path than your loved one who is not going to come back. You need to replenish your lifelines and recall your transports to joy. These might be friends or music or your work or being in nature, but you really have to recall and re-experience them so you do not forget what they were.

Gary: Exactly. Often the act of caregiving can create a new you. A gentleman at one of our Fearless Caregiver Conferences talked about the time that he realized there was nothing more he could do for his wife living with Alzheimer's disease but hold her hand, so he decided to go back to school and learn to paint. Now he sells his artwork.

Gail: That is ideal. Find your passion, or recall the passion that you forgot you used to have when you were 12 or 13, and pursue it with a full heart and mind. This is a time that if you actually do that, you have a pathway to come back; not to an illusion that you are going to have your old life back, but to a new life.

Then finally, we get to the eighth Turning—The Long Goodbye. When you have a long goodbye, you have time for end-of-life conversations. They are really important for both the caregiver and the loved one because you want to feel good about how your loved one is approaching a passage that neither one of you can map out. Being able to bring in whatever spiritual support or religious support is appropriate; if there isn't any, become creative in bringing in people to talk.

Gary: So many of the eight Turnings seem to be about learning to not isolate yourself as a family caregiver. In the chapter of the book called *How to Become a Fearless Caregiver*, we really see how the caregivers we meet along the way have different pieces of the puzzle that we desperately need as we care for our loved ones; yet our instincts are to isolate ourselves, or shut down, rather than to reach out. I am wondering why you think it is so hard for family caregivers to open up and talk with one another.

Gail: The common response that I got was, "I thought I was the only one; I thought I was crazy; I felt so alone and I really did not like the idea that I am going through something that everybody goes through—that means I am not unique." But, I would rather know that than to think I am the only one.

Gary: If you were only able to give family caregivers one single piece of advice, what would that be?

Gail: You cannot do it alone. This is not a solitary occupation. If you try to be a caregiver for a loved one through months or years, even with long periods of reprieve in between, you will eventually compromise your own health, your family relationships, your social relationships, your career or your ability to work, your financial stability, your piece of mind, and find yourself in a dead end. So, the most important advice is to acknowledge, very early on, that you are playing a major life role. And it may be the role that will color your view of yourself more than any other.

INTERVIEW WITH BARRY PETERSEN

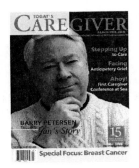

SEPT / OCT 2010

Gary Barg: The thing about Alzheimer's that is so insidious is your loved one is still there, but they are not there. It is the true long goodbye and denial is so easy to do. Could you talk a little bit about how you walked through that process?

Barry Petersen: The worst part was realizing afterward what I had done; and not realizing at the time how people were reaching out to help me see it, but I could not. I guess I am not unusual in that sense. How could it be Jan? She is young. She is really vibrant. She is great. There is no way she deserves to get this disease. It cannot be happening. I think that drove a lot of my decisions, some of them good, some of them bad; but it is a huge part of this denial and this disease feeds it, just feeds it.

Gary: You mentioned our Reverse Gift List concept in the book, which is asking someone not only to come to dinner, but bring dinner, do things, give me gifts. As a caregiver, I need to manage this and I need you to work for me. How did you get that kind of help from your friends and family members?

Barry: Caregivers are people who are incredibly focused on what they are doing in a solitary, lonesome way. Every day, their world shrinks a little more because the person dealing with Alzheimer's needs more attention, needs more care. Life responsibilities keep shifting over to the caregiver side—writing the checks, getting the groceries, picking up the kids, whatever you want to call it. They increasingly fall on the caregiver at a time when the caregiver is increasingly in demand because the disease is taking more and more of the person away. I think people who are caregiving in the situation lose themselves. So if you call them up and say, "Can I help," their answer is going to be, "No, I am fine. I am doing great." Do not call them up and say, "What can I do?" Call them up and say, "I am bringing dinner on Thursday night; go to a movie" or "I am coming over on Tuesday afternoon to take care of the person. Go shopping, go have a cup of tea, just get away." I think it does two things: it obviously helps break the process with the person who is giving care; but the other thing is that it allows the caregiver to step away and realize how he or she is doing.

Gary: I was just wondering, during this process, who was there looking out for Barry?

Barry: Nobody. I was not just in denial, I was delusional. When I saw the statistics, when I realized that caregivers tend to die before the person with Alzheimer's, I said to myself, that makes perfect sense—an 87-year-old woman taking care of her 90-year-old husband, the physical demands, the hours—but that is not me. That is not early onset. It really took our live-in caregiver sitting me down and saying to me, "You are going down." This is a woman who is a retired nurse, who is taking my blood pressure, who is monitoring how Jan is doing, who could really see it. I had to accept what she said because she added something that haunts me to this day. If I go down, if the caregiver goes down, who takes care of the person that you love who has the disease? Her point was very blunt. You take care of yourself or no one takes care of Jan. As she said, Jan will always have people looking after her, but the caregiver does not have that. I think in point of fact, caregivers deny getting help sometimes. Let me go to something else you said which I think relates to this, and that is you use the word guilt. I think in my case, and I do not know how shared this is, there is a lot of guilt that you are not the one with the disease.

Gary: What do you do about it?

Barry: I talked to people who were good at this; obviously, a therapist is good at this. I asked for their help. They explained this in numerous ways; the most brilliant was the guy in Beijing. I went to him and said, "I am feeling horribly guilty." This is after Jan is in assisted living in the United States and I am still in Asia. I am having a terrible time getting the wherewithal to get back on a plane and see her. I said, "This is awful. I feel awful about this." He said, "It is because every time you go back and every time you see her change, you start the process all over again of grieving for what you have lost. It is like going to the same funeral over and over again." That still goes on today. We were out there last weekend to see Jan and yes, when there are changes, when you see that she has slipped away a little more, it hurts. That old friend, that old foe, guilt, comes back to haunt you. So I do not think it ever goes away. You ask what do you do about it? I guess what you do is you cope with it. It is going to be there and you deal with it as best you can day-to-day.

Gary: That is why I like the idea of an appropriately led support group. Even though millions of people go through caregiving, each and every one of us thinks we are absolutely alone.

Barry: I think that is on my list of cruelties of the disease. It is so hard on the caregiver, and the caregiver does not know because you just do not realize it. So I think that to be a caregiver in this disease is dangerous, difficult, and lonely; and, if you do not watch out, suicidal. People do not like to hear that, but I think that is true.

Gary: One other challenging aspect we have as the primary caregiver is, so many times, you make a decision and all of a sudden you start getting terrible flack from people you thought were on your side. What can you recommend for caregivers who are going through this issue?

Barry: In fact, people who were my co-workers did not understand what was going on. Afterward, they read the book and said, "My God, I had no idea!" These are people I work with every day, which gives you a pretty good indication of how clever you can be when you try to hide what is going on. I mean, instinctively, you do this. I do not mean it as a purposeful thing. You just say, "I am doing fine," but the mistake I made was more than that. I protected other people from how Jan really was. I did not want Jan to be embarrassed. I did not want people to think that somehow this vibrant person had changed so dramatically that they should alter their view of her, even though she had changed. Even though I thought I was being honest when I sent out emails and told people about this, the fact is, I did not communicate it. We are now in our third year of assisted living and there are still people who are really angry with me for how I put Jan into a facility. I think my mistake was not being as open as I could have been about how Jan was doing.

Gary: What would be the one most important piece of advice you would like to share with family caregivers?

Barry: Do not do it alone. Do not get sucked into this vortex, into this black hole; because if you do, it will kill you. If it kills you, what good is that going to be for the person you are taking care of? For some reason, we get a martyr complex when we are caring for someone with this disease. I do not know what it is. I have seen other people. I have had the same thing. I can do it alone. I can take care of it. The more the demands are, the more you deny that you are suffering anything from this. It will take you down; and if you do not realize it, then you are going to hurt the very person you are trying to help—the person with the disease.

INTERVIEW WITH LONNIE ALI

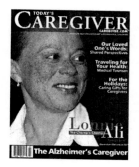

NOV / DEC 2007

Gary Barg: It's impossible to talk about Muhammad Ali and not talk about positive thinking. What role do you think attitude plays in the well-being of a caregiver of someone living with Parkinson's disease?

Lonnie Ali: It's important for all caregivers to keep a very positive attitude and to realize that this is a disease that can be managed. It's not something you have to be afraid of; the more you know, the more empowered you become. If you have a positive attitude, you can put things into perspective and actually become a better caregiver. Keeping a positive outlook on things, and trying to convey that to the person living with Parkinson's as well, is extremely important in the management of this illness.

Gary: It's important for your own health and well-being too.

Lonnie: You need to do things so you can keep that positive attitude. You need to go out and socialize and keep some of the routine you had before. It's important that you realize that you're not in this fight alone, and that there are others who can help you. We're here to help you. You have to call on family members and your support team to come in and assist you. It's important that caregivers realize this, because so many caregivers are used to taking care of people by themselves and thinking that they are the only ones experiencing this.

Gary: I love your Caregiver Tip Sheet. It's so very empowering. So much of your tip sheet explores caring for yourself as job one for any caregiver.

Lonnie: Absolutely. Especially if you're the primary caregiver, because everything rests on your shoulders. If you fall or get ill, then it affects everything. It affects the person you're taking care of, it affects you and it affects the family. So you are the lynchpin, and you really have to make sure that you are well cared for and not feel guilty about taking time for yourself. I have a real issue with that. Whenever I have to leave and go do something, or take time and spend it with friends, I feel very guilty about that a lot of the time. I have to talk to myself and say, "You really have to have time for yourself." It's important that other caregivers recognize that as well. And don't let people make you feel guilty for taking time for yourself. You are entitled to it.

Gary: One of the tips you offer in your Young-Onset Care Partner Tip Sheet is to get counseling or to attend support group sessions. Why do you think support groups are so important to family caregivers?

Lonnie: Support groups can be extremely important, not only for connecting on a social level, but also for supporting the whole caregiver process, and the notion of taking care of that patient. If someone has already been through an experience, they can connect with other caregivers, telling them what they can do to meet those challenges so that they are able to manage better. I would never diminish the importance of a caregiver support group in the community because it's an essential component of caregiving. Not every community has a Parkinson's caregiver support group, but where they exist, they are valuable and it's a meaningful resource that people should take advantage of.

Gary: Why do you think family involvement is so very important in the well-being of someone living with Parkinson's disease?

Lonnie: It's important for the family to be educated with regards to Parkinson's disease because they need to understand what that person is going through and what the caregiver is going through. It's important to involve family members and also to realize that the caregiver is going to need relief as well. They need people to come in and give them time so that they can be away, so that they can do things that they want to do. It's great when you have family that is nearby who can offer that kind of assistance and support to you.

Gary: What role do you see spirituality playing in being a caregiver for your loved one?

Lonnie: You never know why you are given a certain cross to bear. Sometimes you feel like you're in this fight alone, but I think that if you have a strong spiritual base, that there's always going to be a higher being there to support you and that you can always turn to. It's been a very important thing in my life, and in my husband's life, and I don't want to be preachy, but it is just a part of our life; and I think that it is almost a foundation in the lives of many caregivers. You have to realize that we're all here for a reason, even in your role as a caregiver. It's keeping that positive attitude and not letting it get you down, because you never know when you may be the example for someone else; and what you're doing may not just help yourself, but thousands of others. My husband felt that way and I'm sure Michael J. Fox felt that way in his fight for Parkinson's research; and because of their celebrity, they've been able to garner a lot of money for research—not only from Congress, but from private, individual, philanthropic donations. So, you never know why you have something, and my husband's attitude has been, "I work with the cards dealt me, but I don't let it define who I am, and I don't let it stop me from doing what I want to do and what I need to do."

Gary: The work that you, your husband and your family as well as Michael J. Fox and his family are doing has helped to make the discussion so public. And as I talk to caregivers and people living with Parkinson's disease, it all means so much to them. I think it is extremely morale-boosting for caregivers.

Lonnie: Exactly, it is a morale booster, because I know that people look to Muhammed and I, and to Michael J. Fox, to give them the right information and to give them the right resources. It's just a wonderful opportunity for me, as a caregiver, to share with others who are doing the same thing that I am doing.

Gary: If you were able to give just one piece of advice to family caregivers, what would that advice be?

Lonnie: Make sure you find the best Parkinson's specialist that you can get for your loved one living with Parkinson's. Make sure you get the right pharmaceutical treatment as well. Make sure you're aware of what's out there and are able to utilize that information when you go in to see that Parkinson's specialist. Ask questions about what's new and what you can do to improve the quality of life for your loved one.

INTERVIEW WITH LEE WOODRUFF

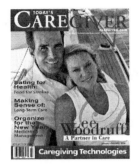

JAN / FEB 2008

Gary Barg: How is Bob doing since he was injured in Iraq?

Lee Woodruff: Bob is doing amazing and his recovery is miraculous; but as miraculous as it is, it was also hard work, as anybody knows who is caregiving someone or going through any kind of rehabilitation or recovery. It is day-to-day and some days are better than other days.

Gary: How are you doing?

Lee: I am doing really well, but I think that we all have our own form of post-traumatic stress disorder; especially when something happens instantly, like Bob's injury. That changes your life and sort of upends your faith in the order of things in the universe. There are moments like if he goes out for milk or something and he hasn't come back in 20 minutes, my first thought is, What is wrong? That is not the way I used to think.

Gary: Has it affected Bob's relationship with the kids, too?

Lee: My kids are much more empathetic and wonderful human beings in the wake of this. Children who go through this kind of tragedy understand how much more precious life is; but my daughter, who is very close to him, gets worried as well. She has been indelibly marked by the whole experience. Children who are in this situation learn lessons earlier than, as a parent, one would like them to.

Gary: Have you found that there can be a kind of joy and connectivity to come out of a caregiving experience like this?

Lee: Absolutely; and laughter, too. Laughter was a huge part of our ability to heal. Bob and I share a really similar sense of humor, a healthy sense of humor. We drew on that heavily to keep him cheered and in good spirits because that was a very clear tie to his recovery, and how much will he had to keep pushing forward, especially in the months when he was in extreme pain.

Gary: How did humor get you through those early days right after Bob was injured?

Lee: We laughed. We had lots of jokes and we called him "Half head." He would struggle for words and at certain times we would laugh about some of those words. Towels were "cuddles" and thumbs were "dunkles" and he just had a whole host of things when he couldn't come up with the word in the early days. He would make the word up himself and we just learned to laugh about that. It was cute and it was funny and it was endearing and we all learned that if we laughed, it just sort of felt better. We used humor in lots of different ways as families do, because I think all families have their own brands of humor, and it was very cathartic.

Gary: When we host our Fearless Caregiver Conferences, we talk about humor. There might be 10 or 15 really funny stories that only caregivers will understand, like your story about Bob with "cuddles" and some things my grandfather would say to my mom.

Lee: Right, and it is interesting, too. Bob was roasted the other night down in Washington for the annual spina bifida event and everybody was so afraid to roast him. Here is a guy with a brain injury who was doing a service to his country in Iraq and how are we going to roast this guy? Everybody sort of touched him with kid gloves until I got up there and said, "Okay, you guys are weak." I just started telling some of the funny stories and the things that we called him, the jokes that we had, and you could see people at first be a little nervous like, Should I laugh at this? Of course, you should laugh and, ultimately, you get the whole room howling. But it is kind of a journey for people who haven't necessarily been there to understand that you have to keep laughing through life. You have to keep laughing through the absolute worst of life because, otherwise, what will you have to spur you on to keep surviving?

Gary: You, Bob and your family really put a spotlight on the subject of brain injury. Because of your dedication, I am seeing more and more information, support and conversation about people with traumatic brain injury.

Lee: I think Bob was willing to put a face on brain injury and say, "This is what it looks like. These guys are not getting the attention that I got as an anchor for World News and something needs to be done about that. We need to be giving them all of our resources and all of our concern." That was a wonderful position to be in. Not everybody would have handled it that way and I can look at him and say that was my husband's decision and how proud I am of that.

Gary: What one piece of advice would you like to leave other family caregivers with?

Lee: One of the best pieces of advice I got was from a very dear friend who told me, "You are going to be overwhelmed with people asking you what they can do for you in the beginning. Initially, there is nothing they can do; but what you need to do is ask them to subscribe to the chit system. You say to them when they ask, "There is nothing at this moment that you can do, but can I ask you for one favor sometime in the future?" It helps you when you need that call made to the insurance person, but you just can't get to it. It makes the people who are trying to help feel special because you actually have remembered and you have called and asked for something; and they are doing something worthy and worthwhile, and everybody is a winner. It may be as small as asking somebody to pick up a pizza, or something larger like, "Can you spend the night with my kids because I need to be at the hospital?" Maybe it is the end, where it all becomes crazy and all you want to do is just sit by that person. You need more of your needs taken care of at that point. I would also say, "Try never to despair." I know that everybody has moments and walls or the black day that you feel is the end of the world. The truth is that each day is a new day and you can look for the little moments.

Sometimes, I would just think about a great big latte with a big foamy top on it. That one little thing might be enough to put me in a good mood for that day and give me something to look forward to. I think you need to take it in bite-sized chunks when the going gets tough.

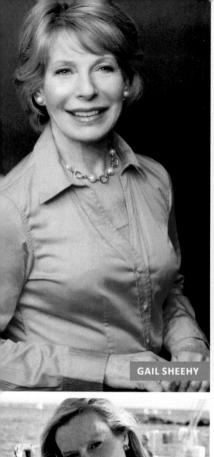

GAIL SHEEHY

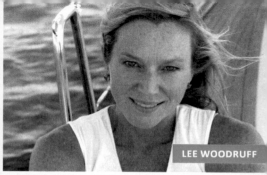

LEE WOODRUFF

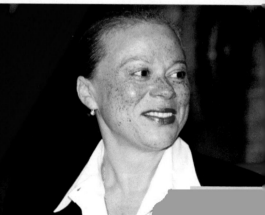

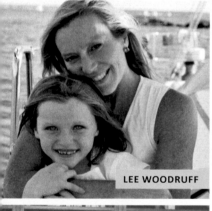

LEE WOODRUFF

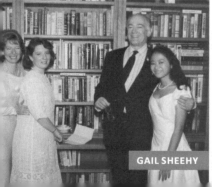

GAIL SHEEHY

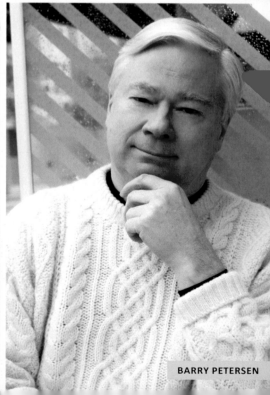

BARRY PETERSEN

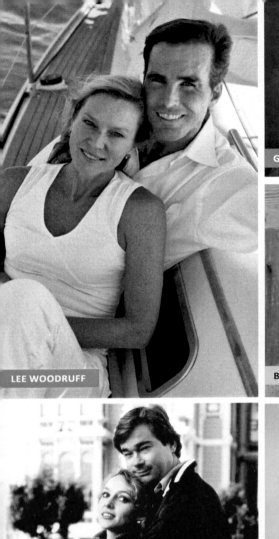

LEE WOODRUFF

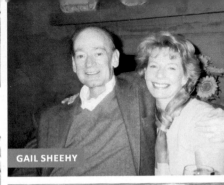

GAIL SHEEHY

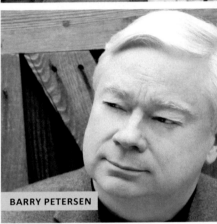

BARRY PETERSEN

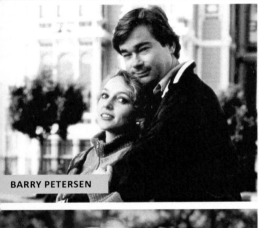

BARRY PETERSEN

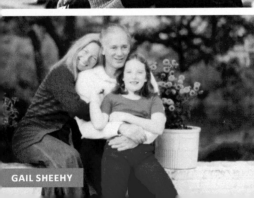

GAIL SHEEHY

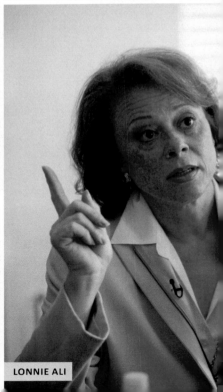

LONNIE ALI

Caring for EACH OTHER

*Never do anything that destroys hope. Whatever the person's
need is that you're taking care of, help them nurture hope.
Above all, see to it that they have what they need for comfort,
because the alleviation of suffering is everything.*

— Hugh Downs

INTERVIEW WITH COKIE ROBERTS

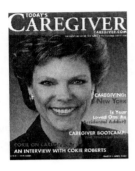

MAR / APR 2001

Gary Barg: Tell me what your personal interest in hospice really is? Did it come about from your role in caregiving for your sister?

Cokie Roberts: No, but I came to understand how important it is to approach death in a positive way. I felt very strongly that this was important to talk about and very few people who knew anything about television were able to talk about it. So, they came to me figuring that the combination of the fact that I had cared for someone who was dying, that I could put a television program on the air, and more important, get it on the air, was a good combination. The calls that come in are just unbelievable. And they've done a very good job of not only putting together good people to talk about the different aspects of death and dying over the years, but also the taping throughout the broadcast is so moving. There are times when you'll be sitting there on the set with tears streaming down your cheeks.

Gary: There are so many misunderstandings about hospice in general and I know that caregivers still misunderstand hospice. What in particular would you like to say to help people understand what hospice really is?

Cokie: It's not some dreaded thing. I think there is a sense that if you call in hospice, then you might as well just call the funeral home and that's not the case. Also, I think that people still really don't understand that you don't have to go to a building called a hospice. They need to understand (a) hospice is not going away, it's staying home; (b) that it can last over a period of months; and (c) that it is a service not only for the person who is terminally ill, but for the whole family. The family often needs a great deal more help than the person who is sick; not only in terms of care, but in dealing with death. I've found often that the person who is dying can cope with it, that they've caught on, and the family is just nowhere near where the dying person is.

Gary: You've said that caregiving is a continuum. Can you explain what you mean by that?

Cokie: That is the message I always try to give young women: first of all, don't think (I do this at women's college graduations all the time) that there is a period of your life when you're a caregiver…When your children are small, when your parents are old, whatever it is. What women do is take care. That's what we do. We do a lot of other stuff, too, but what our mission on this earth is, as far as I'm concerned, and I know I get a lot of argument on it, but that's tough, is taking care. Sometimes it is taking care of the planet or the library or the cultural center or whatever it is, but usually even if that is what a woman's focus is, she's also taking care of human beings; and it's not necessarily just your own children when they're small or when they're having problems along the way or your own parents.

Gary: That's what we tell caregivers all the time. We're asked, "Well, what makes a successful caregiver or a successful caregiving situation?" A lot of it has to do with flexibility and no assumptions of what you expect life to bring you.

Cokie: Right. It's not fair to have expectations of what life is going to bring you. I mean, life is going to come up and hit you between the eyebrows and say "Hello."

And you know, that's one of the great myths. People will say when someone has been sick for a very long time and a spouse is really exhausted from taking care of the person, "Oh, it must be a relief when they die." Well, that's just so stupid. I mean, the truth is, there's an enormous hole in your life after you lose somebody that you have been caring for.

Gary: If you had just one message that you'd like to get to caregivers in particular, what would it be?

Cokie: There are times of acute caregiving, but that caregiving is something you do and want to do all of your life and my basic view is that we should just rejoice in it. Anyone who has ever really thought about it knows that it is by far the most rewarding thing you'll ever do.

INTERVIEW WITH STEVE ROBERTS

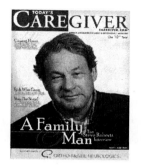

MAY / JUN 2005

Gary Barg: You and Cokie wrote about this phenomenon in your recent article called, "The Double-Decker Sandwich Generation." Can you explain what this is?

Steve Roberts: There's the traditional concept of what the "sandwich generation" is; I remember the moment when I realized that I was in that middle. It was over 20 years ago during a Thanksgiving gathering at my parents' house in New Jersey. We had rented a bus to go tour the historic sites in Philadelphia and I looked around to notice that the oldest member of our family, my father, the patriarch of the family, and my youngest nephew, who was about 6 or 7, were both missing from the group. We couldn't find either one of them and I thought this was the perfect symbol of the sandwich generation—dealing with my father at one end and then dealing with my nephew on the other end.

I grew up with one grandfather in the house and the other two grandparents living only a few blocks away. In my entire childhood, I don't think I ever had a babysitter I wasn't related to. I thought everybody grew up that way. We have all scattered and live in different places; but with my mother moving to Washington, D.C., it's a symbol of the family coming back together—especially when the caregiving responsibilities are growing. I'm fortunate to have a brother who lives here; my father has been dead for the last eight years. My brother and I live about 15 minutes away from each other. The independent living facility my mother has chosen is literally right in between our two houses, so we'll now have our original relationship again after all these years. She selected the facility and decided on it, and made it so much easier on us by doing this on her own. She doesn't want to have the responsibility of keeping up with two homes, the increasing problems with driving, etc. Part of why she's moving closer is because she will be in better proximity to see the kids when they visit with us. This was a very important part of her decision. Caregiving isn't just about the person who goes to the pharmacy for someone, but it's about the joy, the love, and the level of care that a person receives. Care comes in many forms. I often work from home now and I'm only 10 minutes away from where my mother lives. I can call her up and go have lunch with her. It's lunch, but it's also caregiving. These facilities make it easy for people to be able to host people for meals, so this encourages caregiving from outside the facility as well.

Gary: Tell me about your experience with family caregiving.

Steve: As the grandfather who lived with us grew older, my mother took care of him. I had already left for college at the age of 17 and much of this took place after that. The last couple of years of his life, he moved into the Hebrew Home for the Aged when my mother could no longer care for him at home. My mother now has nine great-grandchildren and my mother-in-law has 16, so there is this phenomenon of two middle generations and there are caregiving responsibilities on both ends. I helped my 86-year-old mother close out her home in Florida before she moved into the independent living facility in Washington, D.C., and then the very next week, I was flying out to California to take care of twin three-year-old grandsons and a newborn. We were still in the middle, but it dawned on me that these weren't our children we were taking care of; this is what is meant by the double-decker sandwich generation. Our children take responsibility for their grandmothers and we take responsibility for their children.

Gary: If you wonder how you will be cared for in your failing years, take note of what your children saw when you were taking care of your parents; that will give you a pretty good idea of how your children will care for you. Do you have any words of advice for family caregivers?

Steve: That's a good question. This is going to sound sappy, but I actually mean it. The chance to do this is actually a gift. My mother is giving me a gift by moving here. I'm not naïve; I know there will be times when my responsibilities will be torn. But in these last years of her life, for her to want to be here where I can be a much bigger part of her life is in many ways a big gift to me. Among the things that she did that were so incredibly helpful to me was saving all the letters that she and my father had written to each other since she was seventeen, covering the four years from the day they met to the day they married. This was a gift of family, a gift of lore and legacy, and I couldn't have done my book without that gift. I see her moving here to be another gift. There's opportunity to be of service, particularly to a parent. When caregiving becomes a burden, it's when you're so stressed by other priorities and other obligations that you can't be there because you need to be someplace else. Try to clear your mind and tell yourself that this is important and that the other things can wait. Be there for them; don't be there for yourself. Clear your schedule and your mind.

INTERVIEW WITH DELTA BURKE
AND GERALD MCRANEY

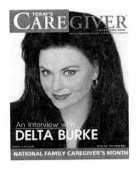

NOV / DEC 2002

Gary Barg: Mac, did it take a while for Delta to see that it was time to see a therapist, or bring professionals into it?

Gerald McRaney: It was a matter of, among other things, searching for the right medication, and just sort of time with the therapist, until things began to make sense to Delta. To me, that was one of the things about the medications that they are not, in and of themselves, going to cure depression; but they will let you get out of your own way long enough that you and your therapist can take care of the symptoms.

Gary: That's right. We're always talking to caregivers about there being no "magic bullet." But everything is a shovel full of dirt for you to fill in that hole you've been standing in.

Delta Burke: There were times, as we went along, he was very protective of me and sheltered me from unpleasant environments or things that were very stressful to me. Then, as I began to get stronger and was able to handle things a little better, we had to readjust the relationship, which was always tricky.

Gerald: And it wasn't just a continuing spiral up and out of it; occasionally, she would go back into a dark place again. So, I didn't know what my role was at that point. Am

I the one who is supposed to be protective or am I the one who is supposed to let her go out and face these things and deal with her fears? Where do I stand now?

Gary: How did you find those answers?

Gerald: You just have to sort of play of it by ear, and deal with where she is at this moment in time as you go along.

Delta: And he also came into therapy with me for a while, where we learned to talk to each other better; because that communication had to happen and sometimes I would shut down. So we each learned the techniques for not threatening the other one, not scaring the other one, or having the other get defensive, and keeping the communication open. That was a big turning point for us that helped a lot. He had to come in for a while, and in just a few sessions, we were able to start practicing that. He would go in and learned more with the doctors.

Gary: Mac, did you find yourself falling into a depression or did you find yourself not caring for yourself? Did this affect you?

Gerald: Like anybody else, I get depressed over stuff that happens, but it's not the same problem Delta has. Everybody gets depressed and, yes, this situation caused me to get into a blue funk from time-to-time, just like any other thing would cause it—a death, a loss of job or something like that.

Delta: He would show it differently, though, because he was very stoic. I've noticed in the last couple of years as I've gotten much stronger and was making sure I was seeing my therapist regularly that Mac started going through a depression, but I don't think he realized he was. I noticed it because there were a lot of the symptoms I had, like sleeping a lot or in bed a lot. I still go back and do that, and each of us might fall into what the partner is doing. I thought, I've got to keep going to my therapist. I can't fall into this with him. I needed to do what I could do and talk with him about it, and then he came out of it. Recently, I had a bad couple of months and I was getting very down on myself, or negative about things. He realized he had to keep doing what was right for him, which was to get out and still do certain things for himself and not get sucked into this with me. We do have to watch that because that's easy to have happen.

Gary: I know you were a caregiver for your mom as she fought breast cancer.

Delta: In '97, my mother was diagnosed with breast cancer and the next month, I was diagnosed with diabetes. So it was very overwhelming, but I didn't take care of me. I took the pills the doctor gave me, but I didn't read anything about diabetes and I didn't change my diet. The whole family was wrapped up in breast cancer. We knew nothing about it; we hadn't dealt with it in the family before. We were trying to learn what to do and where was the best place for mom; everything was focused on that. A year later, she had gone through the lumpectomy and all the treatments and the doctor told me that I'm going to end up on insulin if I don't do something. Then I got scared enough to start to tend to what was going on with me.

Gary: That's generally a prime caregiver trait we have. We forget we're human, too.

Delta: Yeah, you don't take care of yourself because you feel guilty if you do; you should be there all the time and sympathetic and loving and nurturing all the time. That's kind of impossible. Nobody is that good and you can't be that perfect. I remember saying to my mother when she was taking care of my grandmother, "You need to take time for yourself, too," which she was not able to do very well, either. But when it happened to me, I, of course didn't even think of that. You're always better at giving advice.

Gary: What advice would you give to a caregiver of someone living with depression?

Delta: To the person dealing with it, of course, I'm going to understand it a little better. I'm going to tell them that there is light at the end of tunnel, there are other people out there with this, and you are not alone. That was a revelation to me that I wasn't alone, that I wasn't really going insane, and to know that there was a label for what was happening to me. I try and tell people that they're not alone, that this happens to lots of people, and to go find the doctor you can work well with. If it's not clicking, you need to find somebody else, and it takes a while to find the right medication. I was pretty fortunate, medication-wise, because I haven't gone through as many as some people have. Patience and perseverance are a big part of it, and that you are worth it and not to give up—it will get better. That's the type of thing I say to people. As far as a caregiver, all I can talk about is when Mac has gone through it and that's not been as extreme as mine. What I learned from therapy was what to say to him and that I had to keep going to my doctor. I had to keep doing what was right for me and not getting sucked into it, and he has to do the same. As actors, you can never see each other when you're on the road, or you are together 24 hours a day. When we're together like we are now, it's very easy for both of us to get into the same emotional state.

Gerald: Caregivers have to take care of themselves more than anything else. If you become incapacitated, what the hell good are you for anyone else? This can be debilitating on the caregiver's emotional life, too, so you have to be careful of that while you're giving all the love and support that you can; you've got to be careful for yourself. Ultimately, you've got to realize that as a loved one, there is nothing you can directly do about the depression; but, with proper medication and therapy, things can be done.

INTERVIEW WITH MEREDITH VIEIRA
AND RICHARD M. COHEN

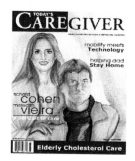

MAR / APR 2008

Gary Barg: Why do you think language is so very important to people living with chronic illness, and to their families?

Richard Cohen: Well, I think language is a powerful weapon. People who have chronic illnesses have a constant battle with how people see them. And I always say, when I'm talking to groups, that you're really fighting on two fronts. You're not just fighting an illness, you're fighting public attitudes and public perceptions of the person with the illness, and many times that can be worse than the illness.

Meredith Vieira: I wanted to pick up on what you were saying, Richard, because perception also applies to the people who are with someone who is chronically ill. We have been fighting the perception that I am somehow the woe is me, burdened selfless martyr. Almost every article starts out referencing that in one way or another when that couldn't be further from the truth.

Gary: Yes, those articles make me cringe and the word that gets me usually is "victim."

Richard: It's hard enough for people who are dealing with serious illness not to think of themselves as victims. I think that you're all but giving up when you see yourself as a victim, and then to have people relate to you that way is a psychological burden. It's hard enough to keep yourself from thinking that, especially when everybody around you seems to want to think it. And I think people who don't deal with illness imagine that we sit around here all evening wailing and beating our breasts and suffering or something. I'm not suffering. I have a great life. I may be dealing with an illness, I may live with an illness, but I'm not suffering.

Gary: How do you keep your communicative partnership going?

Richard: The larger issue in a relationship, and it's so often unspoken, is how do two people continue over years to see each other as whole people when one is severely disabled? How do people who were one thing physically when they got together, when they started going out, when they got married, evolve into something else over the years? How do you see that person the way you used to see that person in terms of being strong, or being attractive or whatever your criteria are? To me, that's the biggest challenge to a couple.

Gary: What about reaching out and talking to others outside of your immediate family?

Meredith: We've learned to rely on friends when we need friends. I think many caregivers don't have a fear of accepting help, but they are embarrassed. They don't want to put people out and are reluctant to ask for help. I think it's important to ask for help when you need help; not to shy away from that. People want to help; so when we've needed friends in times of any kind of crisis, we ask. And I think that's real important for caregivers not to feel that it's all on you at any given time, because it's not.

Gary: I agree with you that one of the biggest challenges we have as family caregivers is to reach out and to ask. People want to help.

Meredith: Exactly, people want to help. I agree a hundred percent.

Gary: Richard, you've coined some really great phrases regarding an area that we find challenges our readers as well. I'll give you a few of them: communication copout, physician-assisted denial and keystone docs. How do we better communicate with our doctors?

Richard: I think that doctors need to recalibrate how they operate. And patients need to insist to their doctors that they be seen in a human way and treated in a human way. I wrote that, too often, we are seen as cases and not people. We are collections of symptoms and not human beings.

Gary: What advice can you give a caregiver or someone living with chronic illness about how to improve their communication with their doctors?

Richard: I think that we shop for consumer items with more care than we shop for doctors and I don't think any of us should hesitate to say to a physician, who is such an ongoing important part of our lives, that this isn't working. I think that people give doctors too much power. I laugh when I hear the phrase "doctor's orders" because I don't think of anything a doctor says to me as an order; I think of it as a suggestion. I think we have to take more responsibility for our own relationships with doctors. I think people are very passive and I think the days of putting doctors on pedestals, hopefully, is coming to an end.

Gary: So partner with your doctor, don't fear them.

Meredith: I think that a caregiver has to ultimately be the advocate for the person with the illness and that means being their ears. It wasn't the MS, it was with colon cancer when at the end of the doctor's appointment, it was clear that Richard had missed so much of it. He was hearing it, but it wasn't sinking in. I think it's fair enough for the caregiver to be there with the pencil and the paper and asking the questions because, when you're the one with the illness, it's so overwhelming sometimes that you don't hear what's being said to you.

Gary: If there were only one piece of advice you could leave family caregivers with, what would that be?

Meredith: I believe in taking it one day at a time and seeing it as a family affair. As much as you give, you get back. I think when you keep it in that perspective, it's much healthier for everybody involved and it makes it, in some ways, light lifting because you're not doing the lifting alone.

Richard: I guess it would be for patients and caregivers to believe in themselves. I think that people are stronger than they think they are. I think that we all stand at intersections or sit in coffee shops and overhear other people talking. I wish I had a dollar for every time I've heard somebody say in any context, "Oh, I couldn't ever deal with that," or "I couldn't possibly cope with that," and I always want to turn to them and say, "How do you know? You're probably much stronger than you know. How do you know you wouldn't rise to the occasion?"

I think that people sell themselves short. People have a reservoir of strength and resilience that is invisible to them. It's something that they cannot see, but it's available to them. I think that if people believe in themselves and their strength a little bit more, the rest can fall into place. Whether it's getting through a bad time or whether it's confronting a doctor, both of which can be daunting. Both are doable; people just have to believe in themselves enough. So, I guess that would be my hope for anybody.

INTERVIEW WITH OLYMPIA DUKAKIS AND LOUIS ZORICH

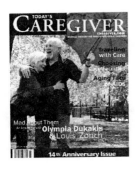

JUL / AUG 2009

Gary Barg: I know you were with both recently screened for diabetes; and you found out that Louis has type II diabetes?

Louis Zorich: That is right. When the doctor told me, I did not believe him. All of my brothers and sisters have diabetes and I thought I am free; it is not going to hit me. But then all of a sudden, he said "Yes, you have it" and there you are; I am dealing with it.

Gary: Well, what does it mean that you have it and why is it important to even know your status?

Louis: Well, I certainly have changed some things about how I eat. Whenever Olympia and I have a choice of foods, she always goes towards salty things and I naturally gravitate toward something sweet. I said, is it possible that I have been eating too many sweets? So I have been trying to cut down on that and a few other things. I have always watched my diet, but now it is almost like I am a detective. I look at everything I eat and I write down what I eat, too – I am very, very careful.

Gary: When you did the diabetes screening, did you do it through your doctor?

Louis: Yes. I get regular screenings maybe two or three times a year; and a few days after one, he told me that I was diabetic. I was rather surprised, but then he gave me some stuff and I am doing okay. But, it was like something out of left field.

Olympia: What is interesting is that Louis paid for all of his screenings. We are trying to let people know that if they have certain risk factors, which Louis had, such as his family having a history of diabetes, his screenings could have been free. We want to alert people to this and let them know that there is a Web site, askscreenknow.com, where they can get more information about themselves and the blood sugar number test itself, as well as what actions they might take.

Gary: Louis, how are you doing with your diagnosis? What has changed in your life since you have been diagnosed?

Louis: Nothing has changed. I am working and I am very optimistic and – is it okay to say I am 85 years old and I am still working? I closed in a show two months ago and people send me scripts to read; in fact, I am going to do a couple of independent films in the near future. I can live a normal life, which is remarkable. I am living a normal life thanks to information that I got and the way I take care of myself.

Olympia: Well, for me, caregiving with Louis is a whole different situation than it was with my mother. Louis is so knowledgeable and so determined to manage his life, to eat properly and exercise. Actually, with my mother, I was in denial. My son said to me at one point, "Gigia (which is what you call your grandmother in Greek) is not eating" and I said, "Well, she is not hungry." And he said, "No, she is not eating; this is not good." And I said, "Well, you know when you get older, you do not eat as much." Listen to my conversation. I mean, my son was trying to alert me to something. And then I finally said, "Well, if you think she is not eating, then you go wake her up (since she was sleeping inordinately) and cook for her and get her to eat." And he did that. She got up and she ate. And she said to me later on, when he went out of the room, she said to me in Greek, "He is a clever boy." And I thought, yeah, he is clever; he knows more than his mother does, certainly. He was not in denial about it.

Gary: You know what? You bring up the three most important things about caregiving. They are support, partnership, and honesty.

Olympia: Honesty! Yeah. The hard thing for me with my mother was just being honest. I could not believe that this was happening to my mother. I mean, my mother was so strong and so independent and fierce. Fierce. And the idea that she did not have control, it was like unbelievable to me. We should be talking about Louis' diabetes, not my mother.

Gary: It is all part of it. It is all caring. It is all paying attention. What happened with your mother was an internal lesson for you.

Olympia: Exactly. And it is also a lesson for me with Louis and my children. I do not wait now. If I see something, bang, I am on it. I talk about it. I am persistent. For example, with all this with Louis, I made it my business to let my kids know was happening, to let them know that diabetes is in their family. And not just second stage diabetes; there was first stage diabetes. I do not know whether it was the thing with my mother or whatever, but I now feel I want to know what is ahead; I want to see what is down the road. I do not want to put my head in the sand like an ostrich ever again. What happened with my mother is that, finally, things got so bad. I was in Greece doing a movie when my brother called me and said that we would have to put her in a nursing home. And then he said, "Olympia, she has got to be custodial." He was the one that yelled at me. My son got on and said, "Mom, I cannot live this way. You do not know what it is like." And he told me about her running into the streets and everything else. I just keep reviewing all the mistakes I made. I am not making those mistakes again.

Gary: That is what we call education.

Olympia: Caregiving is no easy thing. I mean, it is a simple little phrase, but it requires being educated; it requires being diligent. It requires wanting to know the truth. That is what it requires.

Gary: What is the one most important piece of advice that you would like to share with the family caregiver?

Olympia: I would say to look at something and see it, to not deny what is in front of you, to have the willingness to really look at reality. I think that is really important, because that is where everything begins.

INTERVIEW WITH HOLLY ROBINSON PEETE AND RODNEY PEETE

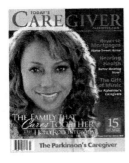

NOV / DEC 2010

Gary Barg: You started HollyRod Foundation after Holly's dad, the great Matthew Robinson, was diagnosed with Parkinson's disease. He was, of course, noted for being the first Gordon on Sesame Street and also writer and producer of The Cosby Show. Why did you start the foundation? What are its goals?

Holly Robinson Peete: The foundation was started in 1997 when my husband, Rodney, basically told me to stop feeling sorry for myself that my dad had Parkinson's disease, but to feel blessed that we had the resources to take care of him when so many people did not. We provide physical, occupational and speech therapies and other services to families affected by Parkinson's disease that otherwise would not be able to access those services. So we are thrilled to be able to continue his legacy by helping other people with Parkinson's disease; especially since my dad has been gone—it has been eight years now. It has been really gratifying in the face of something kind of ugly and tragic, mainly my father's diagnosis. Then about 10 years ago, our oldest son was diagnosed with autism. What we found, among other things, is that autism is pretty much unaffordable, much like Parkinson's. It is not covered by insurances in most cases and we wanted to help families affected by autism as well. So we have a dual mission. We started with Parkinson's, but in effect, it is all about compassionate care.

Gary: You know your dad was in his mid-40s when he was diagnosed, but he continued to work actively for almost 20 years. Do you think that remaining active was healthy and helpful?

Holly: Oh, I think it definitely kept him going. I have nobody else to thank but Bill Cosby, who really could have let my father go on the grounds that it was just a physical grind for him to suffer from Parkinson's and keep up the schedule of a comedy writer. Mr. Cosby kept my father employed and I think that just kept the spark, the fire burning in him. Now, every time I see Mr. Cosby, I always tell him, "Thank you so much; you just gave him such a great ending and he felt such a sense of self-worth." Mr. Cosby always says, "Listen, I was not doing him any favors. He was the funniest writer we had." That always makes me smile.

Gary: What does the Compassionate Care Program do for people living with Parkinson's and their caregivers?

Holly: The Compassionate Care Program for Parkinson's is located at the University of Southern California. It is really lovely because we are able to provide services, especially in an area that is underserved, to be seen by a really good neurologist and to have exercise in their life. Studies have proved time and time again that exercise is really the key to alleviate symptoms and to hold symptoms back. We have occupational and speech therapies as well and we do caregiver respite care. We will pay to have caregivers go to get a massage or a salon treatment, or just something so that they can have some time off. That is so key, because the caregivers are just the glue that holds it all together.

Gary: Rodney, you and Holly have really created a vital personal and professional relationship, but many times we men have a real hard time with caregiving. What challenges did you face when you first dealt with family caregiving?

Rodney Peete: First of all, in dealing with Parkinson's, I did not really know what it was. So to have it affect Holly's dad like it did, what I tried to do is to educate myself as much as possible. From my background, it was the exercise and the health part of it. Keeping yourself moving was something that I knew was right. I did not know how much of an impact it would have. So as we got into caring for her dad, especially once he moved in with us; we got him on an exercise bike and a treadmill. Opening up the Compassionate Care Program really allowed me to understand the impact that exercise could have and what I could do as a caregiver; and the impact I could have just by being there and communicating with Holly's dad and being in his space, talking and interacting with him on a regular basis.

Gary: How important was relating with other family members going through what you were going through?

Holly: It was very important to relate to them, especially when it comes to autism. There was a lot of denial and a lot of educating we had to do with our other family members about both Parkinson's and autism. We were all learning. When my dad was diagnosed, it was in the 80s. We had not yet seen Muhammad Ali and Michael J. Fox and people like that come out and really give us this face and this positive element to what Parkinson's was. We had to learn a lot on our own and share all that information with our families and with our loved ones and get them onboard. With autism, it is quite different because there is a lot of stigma. There are a lot of things that we still do not understand. We understand a lot more about Parkinson's than we do about autism and there was a level of denial that we had to deal with, with some family members, and that did pose some issues, I think that is fair to say.

Rodney: Yes, there is a level of denial with your immediate family, with parents, with Holly, and more so me in terms of autism. Unless you educate yourself, people can tend to stay away, and that includes family members. So you have got to take the scare away and really try to help educate folks on what exactly is going on and how to help, rather than hurt the situation.

Gary: Take the scare away; I really like that expression, because that is what happens. A lot of times people do stay away because it frightens them or they do not know how to respond to you, or they do not know how to help.

Holly: Yes, they do not. Only our oldest kids got a real chance to be with my father and to know him a little bit, but he was pretty steeped into the dementia phase of Parkinson's by the time they were born. They would ask about why Granddad never smiles, and I had to explain to them Granddad is smiling on the inside a lot, but he has this mask that comes with Parkinson's disease that makes it look like he has no expression. It scared the kids sometimes, so we really had to stay on them to know that Granddad is smiling on the inside. Just because he is not smiling does not mean that you cannot smile at him.

Gary: What would be the one most important piece of advice you would like to leave a family caregiver with?

Holly: A family caregiver experiences a certain level of guilt, a certain level of selflessness, and I would just say you have to take care of yourself. You cannot feel bad about giving yourself some time. You have got to have some time to nurture your own soul, because if you do not, you cannot be the best caregiver. Not taking care of yourself is the worst thing that you can do. So in some way, some form, you have to give yourself a break and nurture yourself so that you can nurture your loved one as well.

Rodney: That is it, because you get so consumed. I know that because not only have we been going through it, but I look at my parents who have done that for my grandmother and my grandfather and some other people in our lives. They spend all their time looking after some of the older generation and do not really take time for themselves, which makes them worn out. So you have to take time for yourself, and really take care of yourself health-wise, and give yourself some time and give yourself a break. I think the other thing I would say is no matter if you never hear it or you do not see it or you do not think it is there, you are appreciated and the people that you are caring for really appreciate you. I do not think that you should ever underestimate that or think that it is not true; because even if they do not say it, like I said, you are appreciated.

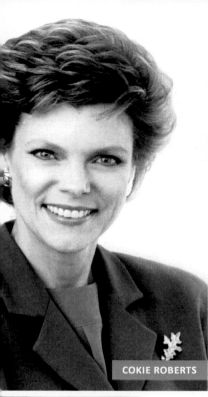
COKIE ROBERTS

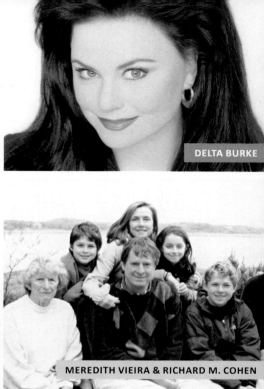
DELTA BURKE

MEREDITH VIEIRA & RICHARD M. COHEN

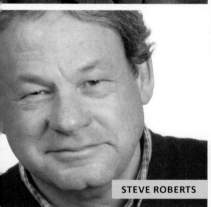
STEVE ROBERTS

OLYMPIA DUKAKIS & LOUIS ZORICH

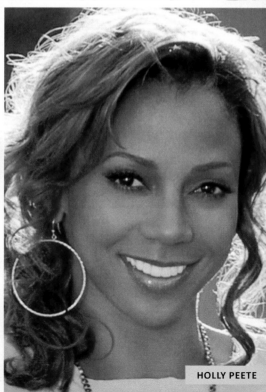
HOLLY PEETE

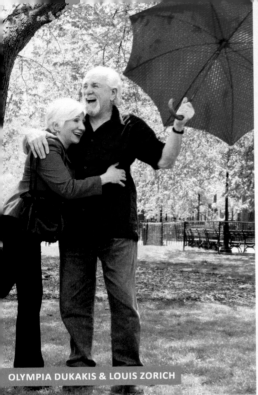

OLYMPIA DUKAKIS & LOUIS ZORICH

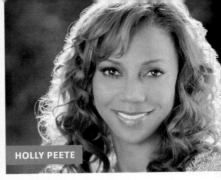

HOLLY PEETE

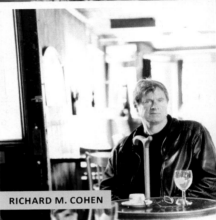

RICHARD M. COHEN

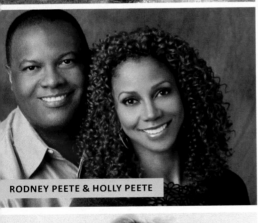

RODNEY PEETE & HOLLY PEETE

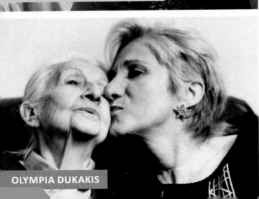

OLYMPIA DUKAKIS

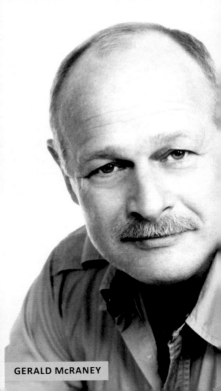

GERALD McRANEY

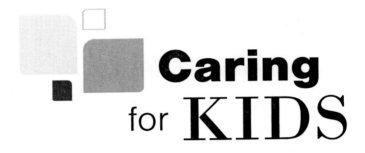

Caring
for KIDS

The truth is, if we took better care of ourselves, then we'd be much more capable of attacking everything on our lists.

— Joan Lunden

▪▪ GARY'S NOTE: CLAY AIKEN

In 2005, we coordinated a fundraising gala in Fort Lauderdale to benefit the Bubel-Aiken Foundation (now known as the National Inclusion Project), Clay Aiken's organization dedicated to people living with autism. The gala occurred the night of our 2005 Fort Lauderdale Fearless Caregiver Conference, to be held in the same facility. The excitement among the South Florida Clay Aiken fans was palpable, and I must say that they did a wonderful job of making sure that the only Clay fans who attended the conference were also family caregivers.

Clay was scheduled to join us at 1:00 p.m. to speak to the conference attendees and we were waiting for a piece of equipment necessary for his presentation...and waiting... and waiting. At 12:45 p.m., I was told by my brother, who had spent most of the morning pacing in the back of the hall with multiple cell phones to his ears, that the equipment was probably not going to arrive and Clay's talk would have to be cancelled—but he was still working on it. I was on stage in front of a room filled with Clay fan caregivers trying to figure out how to share the message with them that their American Idol may not be able to join us for the event.

The difficulty with the equipment's arrival was due to the location of the venue. The Fort Lauderdale Convention Center is located within a TSA-protected seaport and the van with the piece of equipment had been surrounded by TSA agents with guns drawn upon arrival at the security check point a short while before. When they ran the driver's license of the rental facility van driver, they found that he was wanted for multiple bank robberies and both he and the van were being taken into custody. Thankfully, we were able to procure the equipment from another group at the last moment and the day went off without a hitch. Clay's appearance was extremely well appreciated; not only by the audience, but also by my brother and his staff, all recuperating from bouts of extreme anxiety.

INTERVIEW WITH CLAY AIKEN

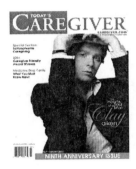

JUL / AUG 2004

Gary Barg: How did you decide to create the Bubel/Aiken Foundation? [Now the National Inclusion Project.]

Clay Aiken: It came about through my experience as a caregiver. I worked as a CAP worker (Community Alternatives Program for persons with mental retardation / developmental disabilities) with a child, Michael Bubel, in Charlotte, North Carolina. Michael's mother, Diane Bubel, was the one who convinced me to audition for American Idol. More so, I worked at the YMCA for eight years, running summer camps and working with different youth programs.

The YMCA I was working for then had a hard time accepting children with disabilities; they didn't have the training for it, they didn't have the staff ratio, they just weren't equipped to handle it. My goal was to try and figure out a way to eliminate all those problems. So, when I got a little more successful and found out that I had more of a platform to speak on, it made more sense for me to try and bring more attention to that cause. The Bubel family was very supportive of me taking their child out into the public. Children with disabilities are known as "that different population," instead of being involved in everyone else's life experiences. That's what the goal of the foundation is and how it began.

Gary: What are some of the things that the foundation has done so far?

Clay: Our biggest achievement is something that we're working on this summer called "Project Gonzo," after a nickname I had at the Y years ago. It is a partnership with the YMCA of the USA, who I wanted to start including individuals with disabilities, integrating them into already established camp programs. We have a program now at the Kansas City YMCA, at the one in Raleigh where I worked, and one in Charlotte. We are going to provide training for the existing staff, hands-on stuff, and include kids with disabilities in their regular camp program. This will be our pilot program this summer. We will advance it further later on.

We also have the Able To Serve Awards, a project with Youth Service America. For years, we've noticed that kids with disabilities are a population that people serve, but people forget that individuals with disabilities are able to serve as well. The Able To Serve Awards are given out to individuals and youth with disabilities who have created service projects that have bettered their community. I believe this helps to take the stigma away from "these children having to be served," because people will see that they can give back to the community, too, and see how productive and what a great part of society they are.

Gary: We are very concerned about the power of language at *Today's Caregiver* magazine. We never say that a person is suffering with, or a victim of, some issue...the disease or illness does not define the person. It is great to see you are helping people change the language they use while talking about children with developmental disabilities. Can you tell me more about that?

Clay: We also, as an organization, try to do the same thing. It's a person-first terminology; it's a person with a disability instead of a disabled person. It's all about changing people's minds. When you start addressing people with person-first language, it comes as second nature. Instead of saying, "So and so is disabled," say they are a person with a disability. They are a person first. They shouldn't be labeled and categorized by their disability. When we stop categorizing people verbally, then we'll stop categorizing them socially.

Gary: What suggestions do you have for caregivers?

Clay: I found it to be amazingly rewarding for myself, but you have to find the rewards for yourself within the work you do. The pay is not great, but the benefits are more; look for that as a reward. Encourage other people to be involved, whether it's as a volunteer or as a paid position. There are plenty of people looking for volunteer positions. As caregivers already know, you learn about yourself when you're a caregiver. Don't just keep it to yourself. It's a reward, so share it with other people; get them interested. When you do that, you get more people doing a very needed job. You end up teaching a person how special this work is, and how special all these individuals are.

INTERVIEW WITH BARBARA EDEN

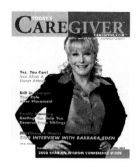

MAR / APR 2002

Gary Barg: When did you first realize that your son Matthew was battling drug addiction?

Barbara Eden: When he was about 19 or 20.

Gary: What were the signs?

Barbara: Oh, there were quite obvious signs, which, of course, I misinterpreted. I thought he was just angry with me and mad at the world, because he wasn't doing well in school. He had been going to school in Santa Barbara, and had a terrible accident with his truck—this was right out of high school, his first year in college. He totaled his truck and lived, and we were very grateful. It never occurred to us the reason he had the accident was because he was stoned out.

He came home and moved in with my mother and me and I thought he was at school every morning. He'd get up, have breakfast, get his books and go down into the valley. And I wouldn't see him until it was time for him to come home. One day, he left his books at home. And I was panicked. I thought, 'Oh my God, he left his books; how's he going to do his work?' I got in the car, raced down to the valley, walked all over that campus looking for him, went into the registration office and said I'd like to know where he is. And, of course, they don't like to give information, even to parents. But, finally, I found someone who would look up the roster, and he was not enrolled.

Gary: How did you feel?

Barbara: Like the world had dropped out from under my feet. I was very confused. I didn't know what the heck was going on.

Gary: What did you do when you spoke to him next?

Barbara: I confronted him, and it was the first time in my life, and he was very violent. He threw things and stomped out of the house, shrieking at me. Then I knew something was wrong. But I still didn't know what. I knew something was terribly, horribly wrong. I went to the classes. That's the first thing I did, and someone there clued me in about drugs. I had never thought of it before. Tough Love said you cannot let him back in the house. You lock your doors. You change your keys. I can't tell you how awful that is for a parent, to think their child, their baby, can't come in their home. But I did change the locks. I had my mother there, who wasn't terribly well at the time, and we waited. I don't remember exactly how he surfaced. I think he was staying with a friend. He had been living on the street. I didn't know that. After he disappeared, his father and I actually went driving up and down streets looking for him. We were out of our minds. We had no idea what was going on.

Gary: How did you know to go to Tough Love?

Barbara: A friend told me to go there. Of course, I belonged at Al-Anon instead, but I didn't know that. This was my path, finding out what was going on, because I hadn't a clue.

Gary:　How did you convince him to go into rehab?

Barbara:　This is a 20-year-old kid who thought he knew what the world was all about. He objected mightily to going to rehab. "I don't want to go to rehab, I'm fine, everybody does this." But he went because he loved us. He was very angry; he had to justify his condition and that was part of it—blaming us.

We did get him into rehab, and he was there for, I think, nine weeks; but as they explained to us, "Look, he's 20 years old; he can walk out any time he wants to. He doesn't have to stay for the full two years." He really should have. We couldn't get him to stay two years. And that's why I think it's important for parents to know early; because when you still have control of your child, you can make them well—put them in a situation where they will learn to be clean.

Gary:　What are the signs of drug abuse that you would tell a parent to look for?

Barbara:　Spending a lot of time away from home, which a lot of people think for a boy is natural, and staying in the room constantly. And sleeping long hours. Grades going down is a huge sign. The minute the grades go down, that's a big red light. People tend to think they're going through growing pains. This is what a boy does. I don't know about a girl. I guess you'd know immediately with a girl. If her grades went down, you wouldn't think this is just a male testosterone thing. People with boys tend to think, "Well, he'll work through this. This is part of his live and learn period." But the minute their grades go down, the minute their clothes are not what they ought to be; there's also a definite drug-culture look to clothes. As he got older, I knew immediately. The minute he lost weight, I knew that he was using again.

Gary: Anything else that you particularly remember that should have alerted you there might be a problem?

Barbara: One of the things I remember when he was just a very young boy, in junior high, my mother, who was on pretty strong pain killers, said, "Barbara, my medicine is missing. I count my pills and I am missing some pills." And I pooh-poohed it; I didn't listen to her. "Mom, you've lost them." She said, "No, I think the boys are taking them." He had a friend who lived down the street. And I didn't believe her. You don't want to believe this. And I know now, of course, they were stealing her pills.

Gary: Addiction is also a major problem for adults because there are a lot of pills being prescribed and cross-prescribed. Many caregivers face the same challenge you did, as well as the same denial, not being able to believe that their parent could be abusing medications.

Barbara: My mother was so careful because she was so aware of that. She had cancer and she didn't want to be dependent on pills, but she had to have them. That's why she counted the pills, so she would know she took exactly what she had to take when she had to take it. That's why she knew that they weren't there.

Gary: Addiction is such a hard thing for a parent to see and really know. It sounds like your first step was reaching out and asking for support through the community.

Barbara: I'll tell you something. I have been so lucky; I had friends I didn't even know I had when this happened. All during the years of his addiction, I had friends that are in the program that I didn't know were in the program. They called me and gave me names of people to talk with and learn what to do. Unfortunately, they aren't all happy stories that these people have. But they're there for you and they're showing you the path. Some of them have beat it, but many of them haven't. And more haven't than have. If you can just get these children early, you'll have more of a chance to make them well.

Gary: Would you recommend Al-anon?

Barbara: Yes, I certainly would. I would recommend trying everything. I went to every meeting there was. I went to group meetings at a hospital with parents and wives and husbands, loved ones who had this illness, and with two psychologists. I think that really helped me a lot. I took Matthew a couple of times. He was not always—until the end—receptive to it, and that's what breaks my heart. He was really trying those last five years. He was just fighting a good battle. I don't want to name names, but there are people in my industry who called me and who said, "Look, call this person; they'll help you. They're in the same situation. Go to this meeting." And I did. Sometimes, it was helpful; sometimes, it wasn't.

Gary: We tell caregivers the very same thing. You're not alone. There are millions of other people who have gone through this. There's a lot of advice out there, but the first reaction so many times is to just hold it in and not want to share with people who can help you.

Barbara: I didn't have that problem—I really wanted to know. I wanted to learn and find out what to do about this. I guess my problem is that I'm a fixer, and you can't fix this. But that's probably the reason I kept going to all the meetings, reaching out, because I kept hoping to find the pill, the magic that would cure him.

Gary: It sounds more like it's a process.

Barbara: I guess. I don't know what it is. It's like you're drowning, and every once in a while you come up for air. It really is very difficult once your loved one is an adult. There is no control. When they're a child, you do have control and you can help them. They have more success with children because they can be kept in a good situation for more than two years. Children have success stories. But once they get older, even Matthew, who wanted so desperately to live a clean life…and one time, there he was, dead.

Gary: Do you have one piece of advice that you would give to family caregivers on this issue?

Barbara: The frustrating thing is there's no right and wrong in this. You're in a fog. You're trying to find the path, a way to cure the illness, and they have to do it themselves. But, somehow, you want to turn that little light on so they'll say, "Oh yes, this is what I want. I want life, I want happiness, I want family. This is better than what I have."

My goal was to keep him alive until he realized he wanted to live. I thought I'd done that. But it certainly isn't easy. This is such new territory. I don't feel that I was successful. But for your own peace of mind, I would say, seek help wherever you can find it. The only thing with drugs in particular is you just learn from other people in the same situation. You learn what not to do, you learn what to do. There are no givens. There's nothing absolute with this illness. You have to realize it is an illness.

There are times when you get very, very angry, but it does no good. Absolutely no good. These people can't help themselves. Only you can help them. You can't do it for them, you see. You just have to support them.

INTERVIEW WITH JOE MANTEGNA

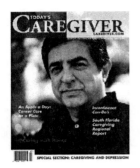

SEPT / OCT 2002

Gary Barg: How did you decide to take on hosting the PBS documentary *And Thou Shalt Honor?*

Joe Mantegna: I'm in my mid-50s, and when I read the concept, I realized it was applicable to my life. It's something that I can personally relate to and certainly can relate through many of my friends and relatives. Caregiving is one of those things that you have to think about, deal with, and it becomes part of the framework of your life. When you're young and just starting out, it's not something you normally give a second thought to. You spend so much of your life taking care of yourself.

We all go through our lives denying the aging process in so many ways. When you get around my age, you say, "Oh my God, where did the time go?" You never think of your parents and relatives as getting older – it's that inevitability that you just don't think is inevitable. They are the people who have been there for you – parents, relatives, whoever, who may need your help and assistance. I do a lot of different projects that are certainly less relative on a personal basis than this is, so it's kind of interesting when there is something like this.

Gary: Then you don't just host the show, but are also a caregiver yourself?

Joe: Yes. I have a mother who, thankfully, is very healthy, but is in her late 80s. It's something that my brother and I are aware of. In other words, I monitor it. I've been lucky in the sense that she is healthy, and as you know, that becomes a big factor. On the other hand, I have a 15-year-old daughter who has autism. It's been caregiving from birth because she was premature and less than two pounds when she was born; and I don't know if and when there will be an end to that, because it's not possible to predict an outcome in autism.

Gary: Do you find that caregiving is becoming more part of your conversations with friends and colleagues?

Joe: Absolutely so. Among the baby boomers, that becomes a fact of life. People are always telling you when you're a kid, people you'd consider elderly, saying, "You're as young as you feel. I don't feel like I'm 90; I feel like I'm still 20." You think to yourself, "What are you talking about? You're 90, you're not 20; how can you think that way?" But regardless of whatever point you're at in your life, you do understand that that doesn't change. We do still have that mind of a child lurking in our bodies, regardless of what age we are. As we move toward middle age and beyond, it's like you start to realize the time passes and physically we go through changes; but mentally, we still retain pretty much the personality that we had as a youth in many ways.

Gary: You have a daughter with autism and you're planning for the possibility of caring for your mom as well—pretty much as a sandwich generation caregiver. Do you think that caregiving isn't just what's going to happen with Mom, but impacts all aspects of your family?

Joe: Absolutely so. A lot of people have different scenarios. Caregiving in my case came from an unforeseen medical occurrence. But those unforeseen medical occurrences can be anything from something like our situation, what you might consider a traditional form of an illness or a condition, to a person who is an accident victim or somebody who had a drug addiction or a mental problem. Anything can happen that incapacitates somebody who you're responsible for and puts you in the position of being a caregiver.

Gary: Did hosting the show make you think differently about a potential phone call in the middle of the night, or did you have all your family planning in place?

Joe: Obviously, there are degrees of planning. Some people probably have more of it in place than others, but I think I have the resources to handle things—as long as there aren't too many phone calls in the middle of the night. In other words, you do what you can within the means that you have.

It makes me understand the anxiety people must feel when they really aren't in any kind of position to handle that call, when perhaps they are in a tenuous financial position, just taking care of themselves and their immediate family. Then, all of a sudden, they get thrown a curve they didn't really anticipate or chose not to anticipate because they couldn't deal with all the other things they had to deal with. So, I think that's what's good about *And Thou Shalt Honor*. Obviously, it will stir that awareness and make people think about the things they need to do, so that when and if something occurs, they're not just all of a sudden blind-sided.

Gary: Do you have any advice or any words for family caregivers?

Joe: It would be that whole idea of planning for your own retirement. When you're young, you don't think about it. You think, "I'll always be working. I'll always get by; there will always be something. I'll be able to pay the rent and provide food." Then as you age, especially when you get over 50 and you start getting those letters in the mail from AARP, you start to realize that you're closer to Social Security than you are farther from it. You start to think, "Well, I guess I should start to put some attention to this if I'm going to be able to keep up the lifestyle I have now. What can I do to be secure so at least I know I'll be able to get by?" You take inventory of your life and your dependents.

As far as caregiving goes, it's that same thing. I think a lot of it is just taking inventory. Looking around and saying to yourself, "What does my immediate world entail?" I've always been a big believer in that. I've never considered myself as one of those people who are on the forefront of trying to save the world. I know people who think in those broad terms, but I guess it's just not me. My feeling is that if I can save the immediate world around me, the best I can, and then I'm at least doing that. I always felt that if people could just take personal responsibility for what's going on immediately around them, the burden would become less for somebody else.

It's like that old saying, that charity starts at home. Keep the circle manageable. Anything you can do above and beyond that is great. There are people who are great philanthropists, people who are caregivers on a huge scale, and they're driven by their ability and desire. I think that is great. Sometimes you may have to pull back from trying to save the world and just try to save the piece of the world that belongs to you.

INTERVIEW WITH JULIE NEWMAR

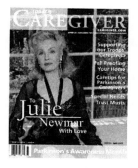

MAR / APR 2009

Gary Barg: You are a wonderful caregiver for your son, John. Can you tell me a little about it?

Julie Newmar: It is easy; it is natural.

Gary: How is he doing?

Julie: Oh, beautifully. He is so healthy. I mean, what a joy!

Gary: That is terrific.

Julie: I guess we are doing a few things right, like his nutrition and the atmosphere in which he lives. I do not know who is doing the caregiving. I think he is the one who is healing me.

Gary: I know he has Down syndrome.

Julie: He has had a couple of things. He has scoliosis, he has seizures, he was deaf at the age of two. He had meningitis.

Gary: You have such a terrific and communicative relationship with your son.

Julie: You know, he does not speak. He cannot tell me how he feels. He does not use sign language. I use sign language with him, but you transcend that. You can read anyone that you love; read them, just as they read you.

Gary: That is what I mean by communicating; you two have a special language.

Julie: Yes. I never feel there is anything lacking about him.

Gary: I've been on your Web site, julienewmarwrites.com. And I have to say with some envy, you are a terrific writer.

Julie: That is what I do now. This is my sixth career.

Gary: I thought there was just so much honesty in your writing. I have been really intrigued to read about your diagnosis with Charcot-Marie-Tooth disease and your use of the braces. How are you doing with the braces?

Julie: I just started. I am in the big adjustment period. I am beginning to get these new legs.

Gary: When were you diagnosed?

Julie: It was in such an offhand way; over the telephone. To tell you the truth, I do not even remember when it was. It did not mean anything to me. I had this long period of denial, or not being there was more my case; like, oh no, no, I can walk over there. And then I found that I was brain walking instead of putting one foot after another. My brain was telling my body how to walk and, through the grace of a lot of charming people, I did and did not know. I still do that, you know; ask people: Will you help me cross the street? Would you do this?

Gary: Oh, they must be thrilled to do that.

Julie: [Laughs] Well, I get away with it; and then at some point, you have to take the plunge and see what there is out there to help you.

Gary: I read a lot about intention in your writings. What role do you think intention plays in your role as a caregiver?

Julie: It is overriding. Intention is where you are going to drive your car and you want to make the trip as joyous as possible. I have never experienced anything but joy with my child. I do not even see anyone that might have a frown on their face when they are looking at him. Of course, you know, I have been in show business. I have stood on a stage. I do not look out into the audience to see what they are thinking of me while I am performing, whatever it is I am performing; because if I did, it would disrupt the quality of what I am doing.

Gary: What are you up to these days; what is going on?

Julie: Well, I am working on three books. I am in my sixth career, which is writing, because a year ago I thought, if I cannot move, if I do not have my million dollar dancing legs—which for me, that is who I am—I am losing the best thing I have. I mean, wham-bam, what do you do about that? And then I realized that I loved words and I like to write. I have this big window which looks out on this beautiful garden. I am a right-brained person, so computers are not my natural friend; but I found someone who comes in every week and teaches me the computer so that I can write. I can reach people, reach outwards to the world; and that so excited me to realize I could reach people like yourself and talk to those with whom I have a real rapport, a real excitement, a real beneficial experience. So, I started doing this, and now I see happily how it is paying off. But even if I did not walk, I could do what I am doing now with enormous pleasure.

Gary: What kind of responses are you getting to the Web site and your writing?

Julie: Ninety-nine percent positive. A few years ago, I wrote a book called *The Conscious Catwoman Explains Life on Earth*, which is very funny. It is about 50 pages of epigrams for when your life goes bad. I give you a little sentence or two. You can cut it out if you like or write it on a piece of paper and stick it on your icebox door to remind you how to perk up your life. I just had such fun putting this together. I call it the very last "how to" book.

Gary: You are a very gifted comedian. Anybody who reads your writing or sees you knows that, and obviously the Catwoman character was always very funny; but that was not how you started out, was it?

Julie: Oh, no. I have always been the comedian because my first career was as a pianist. I had a concert pianist that I worked with and when you learn timing, that then applies to acting and especially to comedy. To reach people, you have to touch them. To touch them, you have to tell the truth that is universal, or at least between you and them. Therefore, laughter is the force that comes from that moment of truth as it hits the body. So there is nothing greater in the God-force, let us say, then laughter. That is at least the second best thing you will ever have in life. Love is the first dominant. There is not anything better than to act kindly in this world.

Gary: Well, laughter brings everything up, opens everything up.

Julie: You cannot NOT laugh. People already know how to do that. You do not teach them that.

Gary: Yes. And truly there are some things that only a caregiver will laugh at because it is an inside joke—you absolutely know what is real and it is funny and it is true.

Julie: Everything is funny if you will allow it; if you squeeze up, get tight, try to force against it, forget it. You are just going to have another disaster. Now if you like disasters, you can keep on practicing them.

Gary: Do you have one piece of advice that you could leave a caregiver with?

Julie: Do not tighten up. To me, the word joy is just painted on the inside of my eyeballs. I try to find that in places, things and people. We have covered it all in what we have been talking about, but a piece of advice—just keep on loving.

INTERVIEW WITH CARRIE ANN INABA

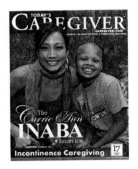

SEPT / OCT 2011

Gary Barg: Can you tell me about the Andréa Rizzo Foundation and how you became directly involved?

Carrie Ann Inaba: The Andréa Rizzo Foundation does movement therapy for pediatric cancer patients. I was working on *Dancing with the Stars*, and there was this woman sitting to my right and next to a young lady who I could tell was undergoing some sort of treatment, maybe chemotherapy. This woman had the brightest light—she just kept smiling and smiling. I went over to her during the commercial break and asked who she was. She introduced herself as Susan Rizzo and she told me about her foundation. I said, "Sign me up!" and now I am their spokesperson. I am very grateful because she is the inspiration. I am only here to help spread the word and bring awareness to what she is doing for the world.

Gary: What inspired Susan to start the foundation?

Carrie Ann: Her daughter, Andréa, had cancer when she was a child and she had movement therapy. She was later diagnosed cancer free, was doing great, and was moving on with her life. She became a dance therapist herself and was going to give back in such a beautiful way, and then was tragically killed in a car accident. It is horrible, but her mom is continuing on in her name and it is a beautiful thing. When you meet Susan, she has a very bright light. I believe full heartedly in what she is doing and I support her in any way I can.

Gary:　How does the therapy program work?

Carrie Ann:　Through movement therapy, you are able to see where the children are holding tension and where they are holding fear. Through types of movement, you can access their emotional state. Then the emotions are released through the session by movement, by all different forms of movement. Sometimes it is as simple as rolling our eyes around in circles; sometimes it is just smiling and not smiling, depending on the level of health of each individual patient. A lot of them come in and they have the IVs hooked up to them. Some are actually still in bed because they have had bone marrow transplants. People are in varying degrees of, I would not say pain, but they are in different stages of their illness.

Gary:　How do the kids respond?

Carrie Ann:　It is wonderful. You can just see the empowering feeling that they have. When any patient is undergoing treatment, the doctors are really in charge of the body; so in this brief moment, 20 minutes of their day, they are in charge of their body and that is empowering. You can see them feel so good about themselves. It is an amazing experience.

Gary:　I bet the parents are thrilled to see joy in their kids' faces, maybe for the first time.

Carrie Ann:　Yes, they are, and it is a beautiful thing to see. It takes your breath away. It makes you realize what life is all about. As great as my job is and how wonderful it is to be on a number one TV show, it disappears. It means nothing in the face of what I see with these young kids—what they are going through—and being able to give them a moment of joy. That, to me, is success. That is joy. That is life.

The parents of these young children often feel helpless. They cannot take away the pain; they cannot take away the suffering. That is heartbreaking to see on any level for any human being. The important thing to do when you are around other caregivers is to help them remember that there is so much they can do in other areas. For instance, in the dance movement therapy, just joining in with their child, bringing their child to the movement therapy class, talking to the movement therapist, and finding out that everybody else feels helpless makes them feel less helpless.

Gary: You have been doing some active caregiving yourself over the last few years. Where is your caregiving role right now?

Carrie Ann: I will tell you where I am right now. I think about three years ago, my mom was diagnosed with breast cancer. She underwent treatment, and I flew out to New York quite often to help her through it. She actually had really good family support there. Her new husband was with her, and he had been a caregiver before. She had a great support team, so once I felt comfortable, I did not go quite as often; but I was there at the beginning, helping her look at all the different forms of treatment. Really, when you are a caregiver, it is about helping the person who is going through whatever it is they are going through with decisions—not making them for them.

Gary: I think that it is important for family caregivers to hear you say that. We always say that caring for yourself is job one, because who is going to step in and care for you and them when you fall apart because you took yourself out of the circle of care and you are not caring for yourself at all?

Carrie Ann: Absolutely. It is job one, yes. You have to take care of yourself because without you, if you are the caregiver, what does anybody have? I do believe that the next role is then to help them make good decisions about how they want to take care of themselves and their future, what medical treatments they want to take, what course of action they want to do, and what supplementary health care and alternative therapies are interesting or not interesting.

It was actually a very beautiful experience because, as every caregiver knows, there is a bond that re-forms, especially when it is your parents. I had not been that close to my parents in a while. By being their caregiver, there are a lot of beautiful moments that happen because you are spending such quality time with someone you care about. I found that to be such a beautiful catalyst, that my mom had cancer. It was such a scary word, but at the same time, so many beautiful things happened.

Now my mom is in remission and she is living a healthier lifestyle than she did before she had cancer. She is much more aware of her health, and she has more gratitude towards her health. I guess her overall awareness of health has changed, and I am grateful for that because it makes me feel more confident in the choices she is making in her life and how she is taking care of herself.

Gary: What was your experience taking care of your dad?

Carrie Ann: About a year ago, my dad was diagnosed with base of tongue cancer—about the same time as Kirk Douglas and the same kind of cancer. It was a very, very difficult battle to go through. They say that this form of chemotherapy treatment and radiation is probably the most difficult of all cancer treatments. It was hard, I have to say. I was exhausted. My dad is a tough guy. He is very loving, but he is also tough and he is sort of set in his ways.

There was a lot of arguing that went on during this time. I thought I saw things that could help him and he was resisting a lot. That was at the beginning because this was a new situation. This was not my mom and I was trying to do it the same way I did it with her. I needed to change the way I was thinking about it. Once I realized that my dad was different from my mom, and that I needed to support him in a different way, things calmed down and he realized that he needed a little help. Sometimes people do not want the care that you are offering, and that can be really frustrating.

Gary: I think that is a really good point; just because you cared for one loved one, you cannot go and use the same armor, ammunition, support, and method for the next loved one because that is a different person.

Carrie Ann: Yes. It is so individual. With my dad, we went through some hard times and it got very scary a few times. He made it through the treatment and was cancer free after all was said and done. He went back to Hawaii, but he still has a feeding tube. Actually, one reason why this was so different was that my dad was living here in Los Angeles through this treatment. He is not a Los Angeles person, he is not comfortable here, and he did not have any other support except me. When I was taking care of my mom, she had other family around her in New York. My dad left all of his friends behind in Hawaii to be up here, so it was only myself and my brother, who lives in Orange County. I felt more responsibility and I put more pressure on myself. Once I relieved myself of feeling that, I realized that it was going to be a partnership between us and the doctors. My fiancé and his daughter, who had none of our family history, were able to just be unconditionally supportive and not quite as involved.

Gary: What would be that one most important piece of advice you would like to say to a family caregiver?

Carrie Ann: It would obviously be, make sure you take care of yourself. Immediately. Please take care of yourself and breathe. Remember to breathe, step outside, and take a moment for yourself. Take many moments for yourself throughout the day.

Gary: That is where all caregiving starts, I think, is to be able to care for yourself so you are able to care for your loved ones.

Carrie Ann: Exactly. The way you care for your loved ones is the way you should also care for yourself. Make yourself the object of your own care.

INTERVIEW WITH MARLO THOMAS

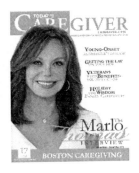

NOV / DEC 2011

Gary Barg: Tell me a bit about the St. Jude Children's Research Hospital and the Thanks and Giving campaign.

Marlo: One of the reasons that St. Jude is so distinctive is that it is a research and treatment center under one roof. When my father was first planning on building a hospital for children with cancer and other deadly diseases, one of the scientists said, "If you really want to help sick kids, Danny, don't just try to make kids better; try to find out what makes them sick." That became the mission of the hospital, devoted to the study of disease in children. We have an international intellectual community and they are the leading doctors and scientists in the world for children with catastrophic diseases. And my father made an important promise to make St. Jude the only pediatric cancer research center where families never pay for the care they receive. And no child is ever turned away because of the family's inability to pay. The Thanks and Giving campaign has helped very much to spread awareness of the unique work of St. Jude. It is the real deal.

Gary: How do I tell caregivers to get involved in the Thanks and Giving campaign?

Marlo: St. Jude is about families. We decided that the day after Thanksgiving would be a good day to start the campaign because the holiday feast is over and families are together watching football games, eating leftovers, and beginning to shop. We thought, why not begin by joining them at the mall? We have made it very easy for people to give. While they are out shopping anyway for their families and friends and spending money, we ask them to remember the kids of St. Jude, many of whom will not be home for the holidays, and leave something for the children —a dollar, five dollars.

Gary Barg: That is terrific.

Marlo: Yes. It is a great campaign because it not only raises much needed funds, but, Gary, honest to God, the big thing is to get the information out there. So many families get death sentences from their local doctors for their kids; they need to know there is a place to go for help. I have met mothers who have told me that they were told their daughter had four months left to live, so take her home and photograph her so you will have memories. But in this hi tech age, parents have gotten smarter. They are not accepting the death sentences. They go on the Web to research their child's disease and often St. Jude's name pops up and they contact us.

I met a father who told me he and his wife had already chosen the funeral music for their little girl before they found St. Jude. I remember asking one of our great physicians at St. Jude, "How is this possible that these other doctors are telling these parents that their kids are going to die, so go photograph them? How is it possible that they do not know that there is help somewhere else?" And he said something so stunning to me: "Everybody graduates from medical school. Some graduate at the top of the class and some graduate at the bottom of the class and they are all called Doctor." I cannot tell you what that meant to me. It really empowered me. You see these diplomas hanging, but it does not say where they were in their class.

Gary: How does a parent contact St. Jude?

Marlo: You should go to stjude.org and search for the name of the disease that your child has and see what we are doing, see what our programs are, who our doctor is in that field. St. Jude patients are referred by a physician; we generally have a disease currently under study, so they are eligible for a current research protocol on clinical research trials. The great thing is when you call St. Jude, they will call you back. All the parents tell me, "I could not believe that the doctor that I read about on the Web site is the one who called me back." We are in the business of saving children's lives and helping families out, so there is not a lot of bureaucracy at St. Jude. Our only concern is saving children's lives and helping families.

Gary: How does St. Jude handle referrals?

Marlo: We do approximately 200 consults a month, even with people that do not come there—who just call up. Often we talk to their doctors to see what they are doing and if we can help that child. Because St. Jude takes on some of the toughest cases, the child and their family often come to St. Jude to be treated. Sometimes the child can stay in their home town and follow the St. Jude protocol. That's because the research being done at

St. Jude is freely shared with the scientific and medical community worldwide. But when a child does come to St. Jude, we pay for everything—travel, food, lodging and all the treatment at no cost to the family. Some people just move in—bring their four kids and move into Target House, Ronald McDonald House or Memphis Grizzlies House. We take the burden away from the parents so they don't have to think about how they are going to pay for it all. All they have to do is focus on their child. My father meant it when he said we would not turn you away if you could not pay. That was his promise. And we continue to keep his promise.

Gary: Can you tell me a little about the programs for the parents and the siblings? That St. Jude also pays attention to the family really says it all for me.

Marlo: Oh yes. Having a child diagnosed with cancer or other deadly disease is very stressful for a family. At St. Jude, we believe it is so important to treat the whole family. We have a wonderful Child Life Program where the specialists create many opportunities for an outlet for feelings. We also have programs and counseling for the siblings and for the parents because we know that a child is not going to get well if the family does not stay whole and they are falling apart.

When a child is diagnosed with cancer, it is like an earthquake that shakes the whole family. But when they come to St. Jude, they start to feel hope. They see that everything is being done for their child and that no stone is unturned and it is done at no cost to them. St. Jude is not like any other hospital where, if you run out of money, you do not get the treatment; you do not get the radiation; you do not get the bone marrow transplant. A lot of stuff happens once you are diagnosed. There are many procedures that may be necessary to save a child's life. I cannot think of anything worse for a parent than to not have the money or the insurance to pay to make their child well.

Gary: When you go to St. Jude's and talk with parents whose children are being treated there, what kind of things do they talk to you about?

Marlo: First of all, they always tell me about their journey, like where they were before they got to St. Jude and what that whole journey was like—how many doctors they saw and the diagnoses they got, the things that frightened them. They usually tell me about that and how they found St. Jude. Then they usually talk about what it is doing to their family. How the other children in the family get scared that they are going to get it, too, or they are scared that their sibling is going to die. They talk about everything—how they are coping and if their marriage is crumbling because of it or if their marriage is stronger. It is just like talking to a friend. It is like being in a foxhole with someone. When you are really up against a life or death situation, the conversation becomes very authentic, very real and very honest.

Gary: Authentic is a great way to put it. The conversations are authentic and real.

Marlo: Yes, they are facing life or death with their child. This is not really a time for small talk. They want to talk about how they feel and they know that I care; they know that I am there to listen. We have good conversations. I have learned to sit there and have a conversation about their dying child or what the child went through and it has changed me as a person. You cannot be the same woman you were before this experience. It just completely changes you, and not just in the way most people say, which is that you understand what is important and what is not important. It does that, of course, but it also opens up another door in your soul that makes you become more expansive. There is a more expansive portal inside of you that can accept and live in a place of this kind of knowledge, to know what it is like to open your heart to somebody else's pain and sit with it, be there for it without moving on to the next thing; really taking part in it completely, moment to moment, without being distracted. There are no distractions.

Gary: It is the reality. What happens after the children are discharged? What is the program for follow-up care?

Marlo: We have the largest and most expansive after-completion therapy (ACT) program in the country. Some of our patients are coming back from the 1960s. That is how we gather the information to improve the treatments based on that follow-up research. In the first years of St. Jude, so many children were dying. When St. Jude opened in 1962, the survival rate for the most common form of childhood cancer, acute lymphoblastic leukemia, was only four percent. Today, the survival rate is 94 percent, thanks to the research and protocols developed at St. Jude. Today, we are following more than 4,000 adults who received treatment for cancer during childhood at

St. Jude. Now that our survival rates are increasing and children are staying alive, we want the quality of their lives to be strong and better.

Gary: That is also a really good reason to remind people about the Thanks and Giving campaign, because St. Jude is a research institution.

Marlo: St. Jude is a national resource. My father made two promises when he opened the doors. One was that no child would ever be turned away if a family could not pay, and the other one was that we would freely share our scientific breakthroughs with the scientific and medical community worldwide. We all have one mission. We are all working the same side of the street—saving children's lives. That is what it is all about. That is why we collaborate with so many research centers and so many hospitals.

Gary: What would be the one most important piece of advice you would like to share with family caregivers?

Marlo: I would say to be hopeful. People cannot live without hope. Doctors can say you are going to die; doctors can say you are going to this or that, but doctors do not know everything. Nobody knows everything. There are no geniuses in this world. I think it is important to be hopeful and to notice when somebody is getting better in this little way or in that little way—to just keep feeding hope. That is what I think.

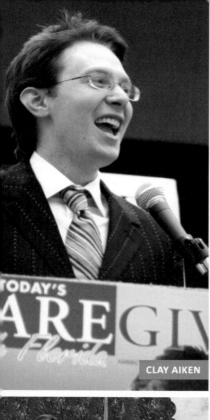

CLAY AIKEN

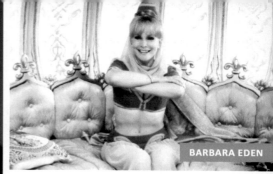

BARBARA EDEN

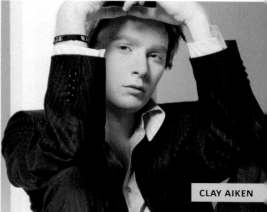

CLAY AIKEN

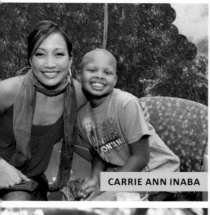

CARRIE ANN INABA

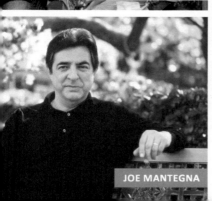

JOE MANTEGNA

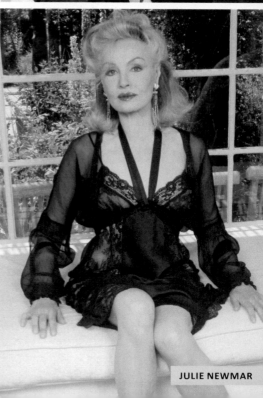

JULIE NEWMAR

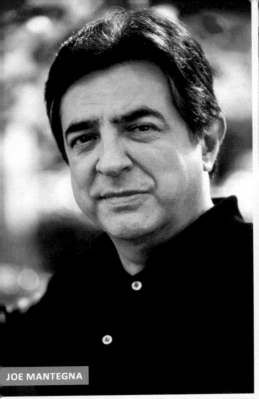

JOE MANTEGNA

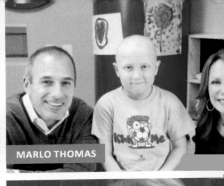

MARLO THOMAS

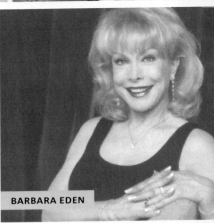

BARBARA EDEN

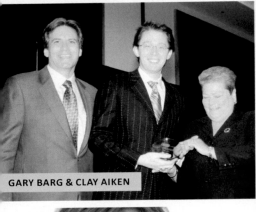

GARY BARG & CLAY AIKEN

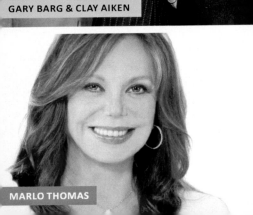

MARLO THOMAS

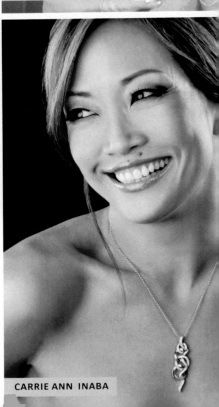

CARRIE ANN INABA

Caring for
YOURSELF

*Give the person that you are caring for the space that they need.
If they need you to be right there for them, then do that. But,
when they need you to back up and give them a little bit of
room, do that as well. So just being there in an advocacy role
to help the patient be an advocate for themselves is incredibly
important.*

— Debbie Wasserman-Schultz

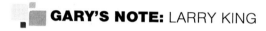

GARY'S NOTE: LARRY KING

Larry King was the Emmy award winning host of CNN's longest running interview program. Dubbed "the most remarkable talk-show host on TV ever" by *TV Guide* and "master of the mike" by *TIME* magazine, the show featured guests from across the gamut of business, entertainment and politics including present and past presidents, kings, queens, movie stars and health care professionals. After a massive heart attack in 1987, Mr. King created the Larry King Cardiac Foundation to provide funding for life-saving cardiac procedures for individuals who, due to limited means and no insurance, would otherwise be unable to receive life-saving treatment. On a personal note, this was the second time I was in an interview situation with Mr. King. The time between the two interviews – over 40 years. Mr. King used to host a radio show on a houseboat across from the Fontainebleau Hotel in Miami, Florida (where I grew up). I remember joining him and the owners of a summer camp I attended as a child for one of his radio shows. I remember how kind he was to a 10-year-old kid he had never met before. Possibly also being kind to the same kid over 40 years later, he told me that he remembered that first interview well. A real pro.

INTERVIEW WITH LARRY KING

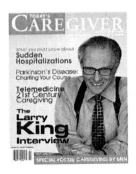

MAY / JUN 2006

Gary Barg: I don't think that you would remember, but this is actually the second interview we've done together.

Larry King: When was the last one?

Gary: It was 40 years ago. It was on a houseboat across from the Fontainebleau Hotel in Miami Beach, Florida. I was about 10 years old and going to Camp Ocala. You were interviewing the owners of the camp and they wanted to bring a camper on. I remember your being so nice to me, and I very much appreciated that.

Larry: That was 41 years ago because that was in 1965. I've been in the business 49 years now.

Gary: I remember it vividly. It was a very good experience for me.

Larry: I remember the name Camp Ocala.

Gary: You do?

Larry: Sure.

Gary: Could you tell me about the Larry King Cardiac Foundation?

Larry: In February of 1987, I had a heart attack, and

subsequently in December of 1987, I needed quintuple bypass surgery. About a year later when I was recovering—I stopped smoking and began to take care of myself when I never had before—we were sitting around and someone asked me how much it had cost. I had no idea because insurance covered it all. So I investigated and found out it was about $48 thousand. And then someone said, "What about people who can't afford it because they don't have any insurance?" So we started an organization on a small scale called the Larry King Cardiac Foundation for those people who have no insurance or have just fallen through the cracks. The first year, we helped an overweight high school coach get a new heart. That started it. Now, we put on two major events a year: one in Washington, D.C. and one in Los Angeles. We have major stars like Celine Dion. Every top star that you can think of has performed. It's been unbelievable. We give the money, and we've helped over 300 people either get a new heart or heart procedure. We help children, people from other countries, and we've donated equipment to hospitals. Our goal is to save a heart a day. The advantage of it is that you see the person you help. It doesn't go to research. It goes directly to help the doctors pick out people who are eligible. We work with various hospitals, and I am lucky enough to make the call to tell the people that we're going to do the procedure for them or their children.

Gary: How can a caregiver reach out to your organization?

Larry: They can go to the Web site at www.LKCF.org or they can write to us. The Web site gives them all the contact information. They write to us or the doctor writes for them that they need this procedure, and that they are not covered for it or don't have insurance. The doctor presents the case. Then a panel of doctors and cardiologists reviews the case and makes recommendations to the board who makes the choice. The process works pretty quickly. We do some of it over the phone. We pick the party and the hospital does the surgery. We enlist the doctors. All of them cut their rates so we can do as many people as possible.

Gary: And you've got a very impressive board.

Larry: Yes, we've got an impressive board. A lot of people work for us. At our dinner in Washington, D.C., we really pour it on. We get a lot of help. It's the most gratifying thing I've ever done—helping people. There's no bigger kick than making that call. Then we visit the patients. Another thing is that if you come to the dinner, you get to see the patients. We fly them in or bring them to the dinner. It's very rewarding.

Gary: How can people support the mission of the foundation?

Larry: You can come to the dinners. I donate the royalties from my books and I give a percentage of the proceeds from the speeches I give. But people can help by going directly to the Web site.

Gary: And people can donate there?

Larry: Yes, people can donate right there to the Larry King Cardiac Foundation. Corporations back us pretty well. FedEx contributes as does the drug company Lilly.

So we have some corporations behind us. The Washington Redskins are very active as well.

Gary: Statistics are showing that 36 percent of caregivers will die before their loved ones do, and I was wondering if you had any advice for caregivers to become heart healthy.

Larry: The one thing you can't do anything about is your genes. Everything else you can do something about. My father died of a heart attack when he was 47. I inherited that gene. My brother did not have a heart attack, but needed heart surgery six months after I did. My children have to be regularly checked. Odds are my children have the gene as well. Now, they have to do what I do. You can't defeat the gene, but you can exercise and stop smoking. I smoked three packs a day. I always thought it would never happen to me. I did some stupid things. I would buy the pack of cigarettes and read the warnings on the pack and that bothered me. Take Yul Brenner. He made a tape before he died. You can see him saying, "I'm dead now. Don't smoke." Whenever that commercial came on, I ran to the TV to change the channel because it wasn't going to happen to me. But it did happen to me. So eat the right foods, watch what you eat, and keep your cholesterol down. There are amazing medicines out there. There are drugs that my father did not have like Lipitor. If you can keep you weight down, keep your cholesterol down, exercise regularly, watch yourself and make sure to react to pain. Don't treat pain lightly. Pain is a wonderful thing. The reason it is wonderful is that it is an indicator. Someone once asked me, "If you had one wish, what would it be?" And I said I wish to have no pain. And that, of course, would be terrible. I'd die of appendicitis or a heart attack because I wouldn't know something was wrong. I react to pain. If I get a pain, I take it seriously. Don't be afraid to bug your doctor. Ask your doctor, "What is this?"

Gary: You believe that people need to partner with their doctor.

Larry: Yes, partner with your doctor. There are some people who say they don't want to bother him or her. But that's what they are there for.

Gary: People are afraid of being a bother because they think it'll affect their loved one's care.

Larry: You're not a bother. You should be there. You don't want to tell doctors what to do, but you have every right to be kept up to date. Ask, "What's happening?" "Why is it happening?" Second opinions are very important. Doctors can be wrong, too. You have to be proactive, and you have to be loving. And, it's very good to have a doctor who knows the emotional side, too. A hand holder is very good, as well as an upbeat doctor rather than a low-key doctor. And that's important because we are all terminal. So no doctor should ever say, "You've got a week to live." This should not be said because no one knows.

Gary: Don't be afraid of firing your doctor.

Larry: Absolutely, don't be afraid. You are the client. People are so afraid of their doctors. They don't want to tell them if they don't feel well.

Gary: Do you have one piece of advice you can give to family caregivers?

Larry: To be proactive—to be there. Don't treat your loved one with pain lightly. Take them seriously. If you have a wife who is depressed and says something like, "I could kill myself," take that seriously. In other words, BE THERE! Those are the two best words.

Gary: Those are two terrific words. I appreciate your time.

Larry: My pleasure.

INTERVIEW WITH FRAN DRESCHER

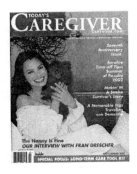

JUL / AUG 2002

Gary Barg: What should people do when they first think they're not getting the care they deserve?

Fran Drescher: First of all, you have to take notes. You have to ask questions and go on the Internet and know what your symptoms may be and what tests could be available. If your doctor seems busy or seems like he's not giving you the amount of attention that you need, you have to move on. You can't be a child. He's not a parent; he's not a god. Your doctor is a person, who is busy, has a lot of other patients, has his own personal life, has his own personal problems. Ultimately, it's your responsibility to take control of your body. I don't give anyone power of attorney over my money, so why should I do it over my body? Early detection equals survival when it comes to cancer, but so many symptoms can be mistaken for much more benign illnesses. People never thought they should be partners with their physicians in the way they really need to be. There are more and more specialists, and if you're not on top of the game, you're really putting your life in someone else's hands, and that is a terrible mistake.

Gary: I think you've been a caregiver to a lot of people since the book came out.

Fran: Yes. I feel like it's been good for me. I feel like I'm really helping people. I went to a fundraiser and a woman said, "You saved my life. I went to the doctor and I felt something in my breast and he said you're too young for a mammogram; let's just watch it." And I said, "No. I read Fran Drescher's book. I am not too young and I insist that you give it to me" and P.S., she had breast cancer. Two kids, a husband, in her late twenties. So there you are.

Gary: One of the things that I appreciated about *Cancer Schmancer* is how it read as such an intimate journal.

Fran: I think that if I was going to tell this story, I had to tell it in a way that's real; otherwise, who needs to pay 23 bucks? We've heard the cancer stories before. But, has anyone ever talked about what it's like to have sex for the first time after having a radical hysterectomy? I don't think so. I think it's important for both men and women alike to know that, a) You can have a full sexual life and b) Things do get back to normal. You can find each other again in a way that's very satisfying and fulfilling. I wrote about it all. I'm a celebrity and I'm talking about my misshapen body and the black and blue and the cruel gash that they cut into me. It's very raw, but it's very funny, and that is what I think makes the book. One of the things I learned from this experience is that side by side with grief lies joy. It's hard to find it, but it's important that you see it; it's always there. People would say to me, "My mother was in the hospital and we watched *The Nanny*, and that was the time we could sit together and just laugh and not think about the misery of what we're going through. It makes me so happy, because those are memories that they will have long after the person may pass on—that they were together laughing.

Gary: That's great advice for caregivers because sometimes we get into that death spiral and we don't realize there's also joy, there's also laughter, there's also life, there's also humor.

Fran: I am very sympathetic to caregivers. I always acknowledge the person who is the caregiver—how hard it is for them. I always encourage them to ask for help. There have been a lot of silver linings that came out of the grief, and I think it's important that everyone finds them when you're in this situation. If you don't get something from it all, it's just such a horror without any redeeming quality. There's got to be some kind of life lesson that we can all learn from something like this when it happens—something about ourselves that can help us in our own lives.

Gary: What advice do you have for caregivers?

Fran: I think that the caregiver needs as much caregiving to them as they are giving to someone else. There's nothing left when you're holding someone up from drowning. There's nothing left for you. You need people who can help you.

INTERVIEW WITH NAOMI JUDD

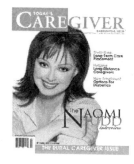

NOV / DEC 2004

Gary Barg: I've noticed over the past couple of years a marked increase in the amount of emails or calls we receive regarding hepatitis C. Is hepatitis C really that prevalent in America?

Naomi Judd: It will kill four times as many Americans as AIDS will over the next decade. I feel that whatever kind of disability God has given me, as an entertainer and as a public figure, it is so I can be a representative for others.

Gary: I think your latest book, *Naomi's Breakthrough Guide: 20 Choices to Transform Your Life*, really speaks to the issue of how important it is for caregivers take charge of their situation. I agree with that wholeheartedly, and think we also become more aware of our own strength. What other advice would you have for family caregivers?

Naomi: When you're a caregiver, you need to realize that you've got to take care of yourself. Not only are you going to have to rise to the occasion and help someone else, but you have to model for the next generation. I've had women tell me that when their daughters see them taking care of themselves, and being defined from within, and thinking for themselves instead of thinking about that silly culture out there, it's powerful modeling. I talk to people about being who they really are, because our culture is ADHD and the media is not healthy or good for us. They're trying to tell us that we're not right, so we have to buy their products. The number one cause of mental illness is not knowing who you are, and you can't know who you are if you don't spend time honoring yourself and living in the present.

Gary: For several years you have championed the cause of rural caregivers, particularly in regards to end-of-life and hospice issues.

Naomi: I helped to start a hospice in the small town of Ashland, Kentucky, because the Appalachian people where I come from have no idea of how to talk about this with their loved ones or friends. I am just such a fan of hospice because my sister-in-law used to run the Hospice of Kentucky; she's also an RN. I used to work primarily in the Intensive Care Unit, so I saw a clinical study for the need for hospice. I'd get really saddened and burdened by what I saw in the hospital. But the good thing is when you say the word rural, it connotes more of a natural environment. I don't know what I'd do without my connection to this farm and any time I'm feeling burdened, I get outside. I have to go to LA tomorrow for the week; so yesterday, Larry and I spent several hours in the woods, where I can literally take these mental snapshots. Before I had to go to the Mayo Clinic and get up onto an operating table to have a liver biopsy, I did the same thing.

Gary: It helps you balance things out. I think any caregiver should take advantage of that in their own lives.

Naomi: There are certain times when I'm at home where I'll come upstairs for 20 or 30 minutes and I'll lie down in the dark.

Gary: But you take that time for yourself.

Naomi: Oh, yeah.

Gary: There's a man that I think the world of, Dr. Andrew Weil, and you are on the board of The Weil Foundation. What role do you see nutrition and integrative medicine playing in a caregiver's health and well-being?

Naomi: Andy and I are trying to get integrative approaches taught in 126 accredited medical schools because we know that stress is responsible for 85 percent of all illness. He had me on *Larry King Live* with him when his cookbook came out, and he had me on to help validate for him. I always try to be a translator for the authority figures, and one of the things I said is that food is like the medicine of our future; when you open up your refrigerator door, imagine that you're opening up your medicine cabinet. There are two parts to this; not only the nutraceutical qualities of food in preventing and assuaging illnesses—and of course we have more chronic illnesses than ever before, and since there are 78 million baby-boomers, this is really an issue—but it's also about understanding that stress is who you think you're supposed to be, and relaxation is who you are. Sometimes, as an RN, I would become overwhelmed; I would look at my patient load and it would look like a tsunami wave. One tangent of this and one of my biggest issues with nursing today is the nurse-patient ratio. When I would feel this cloak of responsibility—and I was raising two little girls at home by myself—I had to appreciate that I'm a human being and that I can only do so much. That was always a real tightrope for me. I think inherent in a caregiver's personality, and certainly in a nurse's personality, is this desire to alleviate or end suffering.

Gary: What do you say to caregivers who are feeling overwhelmed with these feelings?

Naomi: When I spoke at the ANA (American Nurses Association), I spoke to nurses about giving out of their overflow. These gals are overweight, they smoke, they eat out of the vending machines, and I want them to do emotional house cleaning. And by that, I mean first and foremost, if you look at the scriptures in Corinthians 1, it talks about how your body is a temple and you have to realize that the spirit, the mind, and the body are all connected. I want these women, and I think this would apply to caregivers, to know that they have to become a detective in their life, realize what the negatives and the positives are. You have to get rid of what's not serving you. You have to recognize if you have the "disease to please;" you have to have boundaries. Are you a perfectionist? Are you attached to your image? Being a caregiver, you have to take care of yourself, first and foremost, and you have to give out of your overflow. I just got back from New York, and it hit me when listening to the flight attendant say, "If there is a loss of cabin pressure, be sure to adjust your oxygen mask before attempting to help others around you." Now, that was counterintuitive to me and to a lot of the other people on the plane; but if you're not conscious and able to take care of yourself, you're not going to be good to anybody else.

INTERVIEW WITH MONTEL WILLIAMS

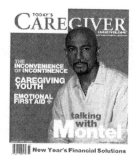

JAN / FEB 2007

Gary Barg: We talk all the time about family members becoming what we call "fearless caregivers," partnering with a loved one's care team. What advice do you have for family caregivers if they are just not comfortable with the care their loved one is receiving?

Montel Williams: This is something that just blows me out the door and I've talked about it in every one of my books. Just because you walk into a doctor's office and he's got a shingle hanging on his wall that says doctor or Ph.D. from whatever hospital, you automatically assume that he knows more about everything on this planet than you do, and that's just not true. If doctors knew so much, none of us would be sick. So, the truth of the matter is, doctors need to respect the patient and the patient's family 100 percent when he gets involved in the process of caring for someone's life. I feel very strongly that if a patient doesn't feel comfortable with their doctor or with the way he's respecting them, or that family doesn't feel they are getting the answers to questions they have asked or information that they need, it's time to change doctors; it's just that simple.

Gary: I always say about being a caregiver, "You can fire the doctor, but they can't fire you."

Montel: That's a fact. One of things I'm really big on is making sure that we take as much responsibility in our own care as we put in the hands of doctors. Right now, the resources are there for us to look up and read and try to understand. You may not understand every single one of the technical terms that are in a document describing your illness, or the possible treatments or the probable prognosis, but you can at least get a feel for what they are saying. This is why you should read every single thing you can possibly get your hands on. I print out what I find so that I can sit down with my doctors and ask them if they've heard about this. They might say, "No, we haven't" and then they'll look it up; so now I know I have my doctors working for me, rather than me working for them.

Gary: I really enjoyed reading *Climbing Higher*. One of the things I was taken with was the challenges of communicating with your loved ones about living with MS. Was it hard to start these conversations?

Montel: Yes, at first; but then the family can make the decision that it has to be a conscious sit-down conversation; we have to be honest with each other. I have to be able to be honest with you, and you have to be honest with me. Let's just say we make a promise, and give each other a hug and a big kiss and say, "I'm promising." When you ask me how I'm doing today, I'm no longer going to say, "Fine." Instead, I'm going to say, "My feet hurt, damn it!" And you can say, "I'm sorry. Is there anything I can do?" Maybe I'll say, "Just come with me to the gym today." At least then I feel that we're in touch, and that you've allowed me to be honest; and I also allowed my caregiver to be honest back.

Gary: I was reading *BodyChange* and it really inspired me to start the 21-day program to see if I can get back into shape.

Montel: That's my life. I work out every day. I've incorporated another phase because I'm 50 years old. As much as we need to be strong and maintain our skeletal strength and our muscle strength, we also need to be limber. I'm now training a little bit more for life and I'm incorporating a lot more stretching.   I'll be incorporating a lot more yoga and a lot of other forms of exercise, along with my resistance training and my agility training.   I'm doing all these things together, so I focus on that. I'm in the process of writing my next book; not only addressing eating, but also being fit for life.

Gary: What would you say a family caregiver needs to do to start incorporating exercise into their life?

Montel: Of course, check with a doctor first; but the thing you need to do is to start with something simple. As crazy as it sounds, take a walk. Forget the weights, the gym, and the trainer; go out the front door and take a walk. The first time, walk until you feel tired, but know you can get back to your house. The next day, walk until you get tired and tell yourself, "I'm just going to go three more minutes." Then, the next time, you look at your watch. If it's the same time you got tired the day before, go six more minutes. The next time you go, I guarantee you that it will not be the same time as before. You've achieved something. That's called physical exercise, right there; that's your first achievement. If you've done this, then you're ready to start on an exercise program by increasing that walking. One of the things people think to get in shape is that you've got to do it tomorrow because there's something so action-oriented about "get in shape." It sounds almost as if it were an order, to do it right now. The truth is, even if you attempted to do it right now, it takes time; so take the pressure off yourself and recognize that it takes time. You have to find those little things that get you down the path of feeling like you've accomplished something, and the quickest way to accomplish this is by walking out your front door. A lot of times we look at this as "I have to get to the gym" or "I have to go to the mall to get an outfit and I have to look cute while exercising and I've got to get my make up on" and so they never end up walking out the door.

Gary: I've been reading a lot about the Montel Williams MS Foundation. Can you tell me about the work of the foundation?

Montel: I started this foundation right after my diagnosis. I kept hearing about all the money being raised all over the world to find a cure, and I was finding out that a lot of that money wasn't really going to cures; it was going to the salaries and buildings and monuments of people rather than curing the disease. I wanted to start a foundation where 100 percent of the money donated and earmarked for research to find a cure went exactly there. So, the Montel Williams MS Foundation was established to find a cure, educate the public on the disease, and once we find a cure, see if we can provide medication to those who can't afford it. To date, we've given about a million dollars to some of the top hospitals around the world. Two of the projects that we're very, very proud of are at the Karolinska Institute of Stockholm, Sweden. One is being conducted by Dr. Tomas Olsen, for having found two of the genes that seem to not only be the catalyst for MS, but also for rheumatoid arthritis and for a heart malady. We also have a doctor who is working on a stem cell project. They have actually created spinal cord tissue; and if that's true, the implications four or five years from now could be profound when it comes to MS or other illnesses where there's damage being done to the spinal cord or brain matter. We've also helped in the development of what now may be the first blood test for MS.

Gary: What would be the one piece of advice you'd like family caregivers to take from this interview?

Montel: Caregivers have to understand that God blesses you for what you do, but if you don't stop every now and then to take care of yourself, you won't do any good for anybody. The person you're taking care of won't be able to absorb your humanity or your spirit if you're depressed, if you yourself are tired, if you aren't paying attention to your own personal health. The one thing that I think is really important for all caregivers to understand is that every now and then, it goes back to that thought of being honest with the person and building an honest relationship with that person; do not be afraid to speak without offending. There may come a moment when you have to tell your friend that I love you, but I need a little break, and I bet you could use a little break from me, too, so let me take one and I'll see you in a few hours or in a few days. Take a break, rather than let it fester and damage your relationship.

INTERVIEW WITH HELEN REDDY

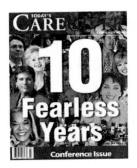

MAY / JUN 2008

Gary Barg: I know you retired from performing in 2002 and now are a practicing hypnotherapist. What caused the change in your career?

Helen Reddy: I had been in show business for nearly 55 years, since I was five years old. I wanted to do something else and hypnotism was a lifelong interest.

Gary: You explore the evolution of that transition in your book. What made you decide to write it?

Helen: I had been asked many times over the years if I would write an autobiography, and I really did not have any interest because they were stressing, "Tell us all about sex, drugs, and rock and roll" so to speak. That was not really my life.

But, I was already doing the hypnotherapy and I was living on Norfolk Island when I got a call from the hospital saying that the psychiatrist was visiting and he wanted to meet me before he referred patients to me.

So, I went down to the hospital and I met him and it was very serendipitous. His office was in the building at the end of the street where my sister lived. It turned out that we had a lot of mutual friends. His wife was on the island with him and she was the literary agent for my daughter's godfather. Her brother was with them. He lived on the street I grew up on. There were all these connections.

I had dinner with him, his wife and her brother and about a month later, she sent me a whole pile of books that she had either written or edited or published herself with a note saying, "Would you be interested in doing a body, mind, spirit book?" We had talked a lot about psychic things during the dinner. I thought about it and decided, "Well, yes, that is a book I would be interested in writing."

And so, I set about writing it and I found that I needed to place the experiences that I had had in the context of my life. I needed to show the growth and the progression and all the things that surrounded those areas. Before I knew what I was doing, I was writing a memoir.

Gary: What is fascinating is that it weaves your professional career with the things you had discovered even as a child. I think you had your first out of body experience when you were a young girl. What was that like?

Helen: At first, I thought I had died because I was out of my body. I was looking at my body and my face. I am lying there and I thought I had died. That was kind of traumatic. But at the same time, there was the realization that life does go on; that we are simply inside a body. In other words, I was not the body; I was somebody who had been in that body. And so that raised a lot of issues with me because I had not been able to get too many of my questions answered by religion, and I actually became an atheist at age nine. Having that experience at age 11 really brought me back to spirituality and led me on a lifelong search. I learned about reincarnation in the mid-fifties. There was a book called *The Search for Bridey Murphy* and that was fascinating. I did not know anything about reincarnation, but now here was an explanation for so many of the things that religion could not give me an answer for. Having grown up in show business, I had seen stage hypnotists; but I had never thought that maybe hypnotism could be a tool for research, nor did I have any idea that 50 years later it would be an accepted branch of science and I would practicing it.

Gary: The thought about reincarnation, about past life, about all of us being on a path has to be comforting to somebody who has a loved one at the end of their life.

Helen: Oh, definitely, and to the loved ones themselves, too, you know? That life does continue. I believe that we are consciousness, consciousness is energy, and energy can never be destroyed. It can be transformed, but it can never be destroyed.

Gary: What benefit would you think that caregivers might have from the services of a hypnotherapist?

Helen: I have a dear friend in Sydney. Her husband has Alzheimer's. He is in his nineties now and she could not manage him at home anymore; but she faithfully sees him every day, and has every meal with him, but she herself is pretty much at the end of her rope. I have said to her, "Please come and see me because one hour of hypnotherapy equals eight hours sleep and I would really like to give you some relief for what you are going through." I think it can be tremendously helpful, just purely from a relaxation point of view, that somebody get to set aside their gear and go to another place.

Gary: You have Addison's disease. But, I also know that you had to fight with the medical community for an accurate diagnosis and it is something we go through as caregivers a lot. Do you have any advice for caregivers who do not think they are really getting the help they need?

Helen: The problem with Addison's is it is such a rare disease. When I first went to Norfolk Island, there were three resident doctors and one of them took me into the room where they all meet. He said, "I want you to meet someone with Addison's disease" because none of them had ever met anybody with it so the symptoms can be confusing. Two patients can have totally different sets of symptoms. We have all heard stories where doctors have simply misdiagnosed or not known what it was or accused us of malingering.

Gary: A lot of different diseases manifest themselves in ways that the health care system will pretty much just brush you off saying they know better. What did it take for you to keep pushing through to get the answers you were looking for?

Helen: I was being given placebos, and the doctor told my husband at the time that I should see a psychiatrist because I was convinced that there was something wrong with me. Then I happened to meet Dr. Georgie who has since passed on. She had seen it before. She had actually been the one, I think, who had diagnosed JFK. So, as soon as I told her that I had a kidney removed when I was in my teens, she said, "Did they take out the adrenal gland?" And I said, "Well, I have no idea." But she ordered all these tests and within four days, there was the diagnosis. Not only that, as soon as I was on cortisone, there was an immediate difference. I mean, I was back to feeling normal again. I remember when I first went in there, she said, "So, you feel sick?" I said, "No, I do not feel sick. I just do not feel well." She said, "Then something is wrong. Let us find out what it is."

Gary: I think reading your book, and reading about what you have been through, that there is definitely a message for people not to think, "This is it. I am in this life. I am dealing with this. I am suffering and there is nothing before, there is nothing after, and there is nothing I can do about it."

Helen: You are talking about the feeling of helplessness. That is difficult. But look, you can only take one day at a time. I find caregivers are very reluctant to ask for help. But I think sometimes you just have to reach out and say, "Look, I really need a day off. Can you possibly take care of my responsibilities for an afternoon?" or something along those lines because you have to fill the well.

Gary: Would you have one piece of advice that you would like to leave with family caregivers?

Helen: I would stress that life is eternal, that love never dies.

INTERVIEW WITH BARRY MANILOW

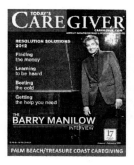

JAN / FEB 2012

Gary Barg: Watching you perform, it is hard to believe that you were dealing with atrial fibrillation (A-fib) even while you were on stage. How did the disease manifest itself and what did you do?

Barry Manilow: About 15 years ago, I was driving home and it felt to me like my heart skipped a beat, which did not seem very important. But as I kept driving, my heart skipping a beat kept getting more and more out of whack. It was not just a little skipping a beat; it started to feel like it was—the only way I can put it is out of rhythm.

Your heart goes faster when you are jogging or when you are excited. You hear a boom-boom-boompa-dum and maybe it goes faster—boompa-doompa-doomp; it's the same tempo. But with A-fib, it goes out of whack—ba-doomp-boom, badooma-dooma-dooma-badooma-badooma wumpadoomp—like that. The first time it happened, I thought, well, I am dying or something. What's going on here? And then it kind of went away and I did not do anything about it, which was wrong.

It came back about a week later. It is kind of insidious in that it does not come from stress, or from being excited; it does not come from anything. It just starts when it wants to start. I think I was watching television. I could feel my heart start to do that same thing; it was going out of rhythm again.

That is when I called my doctor and he knew exactly what I was talking about. He said, "You have got atrial fibrillation," and described exactly what I had and gave me medication. It could have stopped right there. That is why I tell people, "Go see your doctor." If you feel what I am talking about, if this sounds familiar to you, go to your doctor. That is what you need to do. You need to have a dialog and a relationship with your doctor so that you know whether it is getting worse or whether it is calming down and what medication he can put you on; you can live a very normal life. Just by having the doctor treat you with simple medication, it could stop right there for you. With me, it did not stop right there and with a lot more people, it did not stop right there.

Garg: You have mentioned the word "rhythm"; it leads to my next question of what is the "Get Back in Rhythm" campaign?

Barry: To make people aware of this condition, this atrial fibrillation. As you go on GetBackinRhythm.com, they have put together what I am trying to say, only much more articulately, and they have a little test – "Do you have this? Does it feel like this?" If you check off enough boxes, then you know you probably have atrial fibrillation and you need to get yourself to a doctor.

Gary: That is good to know. Frankly, as family caregivers, we take ourselves out of this circle of care. We ignore our own issues; and then I always tell caregivers if you do that, who is going to step in and care for you and your loved one? This sounds dangerous.

Barry: You are right. It is dangerous. I have spoken to many doctors and they say, "So many people do not like to go to their doctors." One doctor said, "You are like me; I do not like to go to doctors." And he was a doctor! It is very common. But with this one, you really have to take it seriously because it can go to some really nasty places.

Garg: Pretty quickly, too.

Barry: Once the medication stops working, as it does with me, I cannot stop my heart from going crazy. Then they have to stop it because you are playing with fire if they don't. They give you what is called cardio aversion. They give you the paddles—I call them paddles—what we have seen on TV all the time where they say, "Clear!" and then bang!—those paddles. They put you out so you do not really feel very much. It is terrifying, but when you wake up, your heart is back in rhythm. That is when the medication does not work; that is the next step. They have to do something as dramatic as that because they have got to stop it somehow. They have cardio averted me—they have given me the paddles—I cannot even remember how many times over 15 years.

Garg: Now you know what to do about A-fib and, obviously, cardio aversion; how else does it affect your life?

Barry: It is a pain in the neck. It comes on in the middle of an interview like you and I are having. It comes on in the middle of my life. It never really has come on when I have been in the wings waiting to go on stage. I do not know why; it has just left me alone on that.

But there was one time when I was in Boston. I was in a thing with the Boston Philharmonic on July 4th. It was a live TV show being broadcast to millions of people. I woke up in the morning and I felt this thing start. I went, "Oh no, not now, please." I took the medicine the way I was supposed to and it just would not stop. I called my doctor and said, "Okay, what do I do? I have a sound check at 2 o'clock." This was around 9 o'clock in the morning. He said, "Get over to the hospital in Boston; there is an area that is devoted to A-fib." I got myself a doctor there and they knew who I was; they got me in. Sure enough; they had to stop it with the paddles.

After it was done, I woke up and the thing had stopped. I went to sound check and kind of staggered onto the stage. Nobody knew and that night I did the show. You can get through your life, but you have got to take care of yourself; that is it. You have got to be on top of it.

Garg: I have seen you perform live and I was thinking about this because you bring so much to the stage; you have so much energy. I was wondering if you are worried about that happening in the middle of the performance.

Barry: I think if it did happen, I could get through the performance. It does not stop me from living my life. Most of the time, the medication does its job and pulls it all back together again. But sometimes even that does not work. I have not had any episodes while I have been on stage.

Garg: That is great. Do they tell you to restrict exercise or do different exercises?

Barry: No. Many people ask what I do; there are no rules—everybody is different. For some people, there is caffeine and in other people, it is too much exercise. It just goes—everybody has got a different reason—do not eat this kind of thing, do not drink that kind of thing. For me, no one has ever told me not to do this or that. I just take the medication and go on with my life. If I had not gone to the doctor, I do not know if I could have easily gone on with my life.

Gary: I think that is the key. It sounds like when you feel that irregular rhythm that mostly just comes out of the blue, do not ignore it; get medical help.

Barry: Not just that one time. You have got to form a relationship with your doctor because just going to your doctor once is not the answer. Because if you have got it, it is not going away; there is no cure for this. You have got to call him when you feel it is coming on and know that he is on the other end of the phone when you need him.

Gary: We call it a partnership.

Barry: A partnership. That is a good one; form a partnership with your doctor.

Gary: What would you think is the one most important piece of advice you would like to share with family caregivers about A-fib?

Barry: You have got to take this one seriously. It comes on very innocently. I can understand why people would say other people have worse problems than I do. I do not think that is a good way to deal with this. If anybody is reading this interview and it sounds familiar to them, you have got to take it seriously because, like I said, you are playing with fire. If you say that my family has got more problems, well, if you do not take care of this, you are going to be a big problem in your family.

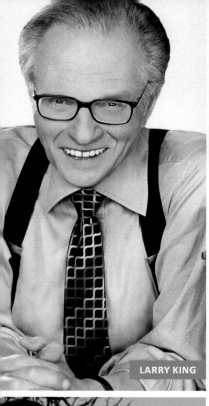

LARRY KING

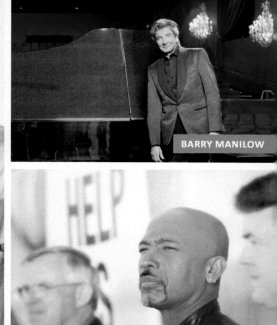

BARRY MANILOW

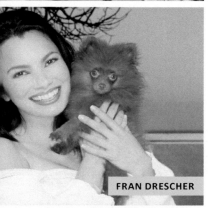

FRAN DRESCHER

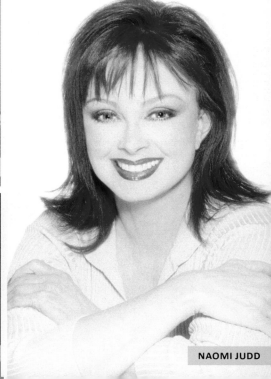

MONTEL WILLIAMS

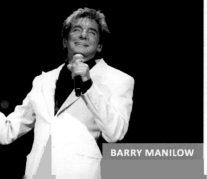

BARRY MANILOW

NAOMI JUDD

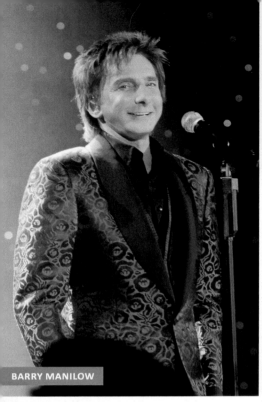

BARRY MANILOW

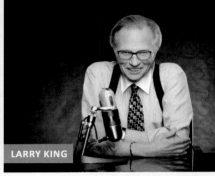

LARRY KING

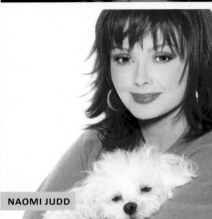

NAOMI JUDD

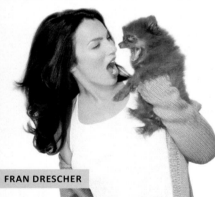

FRAN DRESCHER

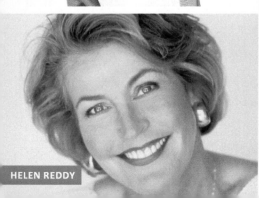

HELEN REDDY

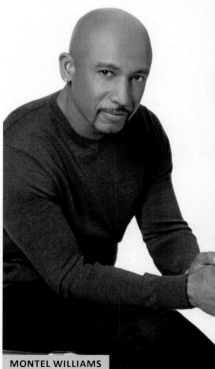

MONTEL WILLIAMS

In MEMORIUM

Dana was an amazing woman. Chris and Dana, to this day, are my inspiration. Chris could very easily have focused on what he needed to make his life more comfortable. Instead, he went out of his way and pushed himself to the limit to try and find a cure and work for other people with disabilities. And Dana was a tirelessly wonderful caregiver.

— Jane Seymour

GARY'S NOTE: DANA REEVE

In 1998, I received a call from an upcoming cover interview subject who took a break from helping her parents move into a new home to speak with me. After Dana Reeve finished our interview, she went right back to moving boxes and furniture for her mom and dad. Through the years, we all came to know Dana because of her family's personal story of courage and her commitment throughout Chris' injury, the creation of the Christopher Reeve Paralysis Foundation and his passing.

One of the most striking things about Dana was her absolute honesty. I have quoted from her interview many times in conferences and private conversations with caregivers. She was so frank and open, that at first I wondered if she knew that I was writing everything down for the interview. But as I came to learn, these qualities characterized just who she was as a person. I think it is important to remember Dana Reeve as more than just a dedicated activist and/or as the wife of Christopher Reeve. She was a loving mother and daughter, a terrific singer and actress, and she gave me lots of material for my speeches over the years. She spoke of the need for caregivers to take "a mental bubble bath," getting friends and family members to help as you deal with the healthcare system, finding wisdom from other family caregivers, and how to best work with insurance companies. She was a true caregiving expert and advocate.

INTERVIEW WITH DANA REEVE

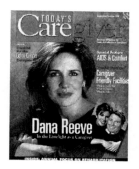

SEPT / OCT 1998

Gary Barg: How did you explain to your son, Will, about his father's accident?

Dana Reeve: As a parent, I firmly believe that we need to be as honest as we can be with our children, tempering what we say to match the appropriate age level of the child. Children are extremely resilient. I think if they feel safe, then you're giving them the best possible tool any parent would give a child: to be able to cope with life's inevitable difficulties.

At first, Will (he was three years old) was afraid of even seeing Chris, but he adapted very quickly. Will repeatedly fell off his hobby horse in the pediatric ward playroom and would say, "Oh, my neck, my neck!" I would have to tell him that his neck was fine and "Daddy's neck is broken and he can't move." We would do this over and over again. It was sort of like play therapy that he was devising on his own.

Gary: How have the past three years changed your perspective on life?

Dana: Oh, boy, I don't take anything for granted. I'm also more cynical and more pragmatic. I don't take a romantic view of life at all anymore; I really take a practical view of life. I don't necessarily see that as a loss, but I do see it as a difference. "Happily ever after," is like, "Ha-ha-ha." However, the other side of that is entering into a world where you see the gift behind disability. I mean, it's not as frivolous. There's an intensity to life and relationships which in many ways is extremely fulfilling. I think there's a lot of truth to the adage, "What doesn't kill you makes you stronger." I'm also finding that you can find joy in the oddest of places and activities.

Gary: Like what?

Dana: Just in small things. We were looking at the stars the other night, and the idea that Chris can be out of bed, and the stars were out, and it was so clear with the most beautiful breeze. You just appreciate you're alive, and you're able to look at the stars, and everybody is healthy at the moment. I think that helps us appreciate our family relationship even more.

Gary: What has helped you get through these times?

Dana: Therapy. I'm a big believer in therapy if you have someone very, very good and qualified. There are some things that I don't think are helpful to share with your spouse. I do think a bad therapist is worse than none at all, but there are wonderful clinical psychologists out there. I consider it to be similar to getting a heart doctor for your heart. A therapist is an emotion doctor for your emotions.

Gary: How do you deal with stress?

Dana: Stress is an ongoing problem. I find yoga is really helpful, but then I find my life gets so stressed out, I don't have time for yoga. No time for the cure. It's ironic; one of the things I speak on is nurturing the nurturer. I really believe in it. I was telling a friend of mine that I was going to speak on it, and she looked at me and said, "Better start practicing what you preach." I do think you can deal with stress in little ways, you can give yourself little getaways, and it doesn't always have to cost money. It's really a gift you have to give yourself: mini respites.

Gary: What do you do for your "mini respites"?

Dana: Yoga is great when I take the time. But even when I don't, I would just go up into a room where no one will come in and do whatever it takes, whether it's reading, sitting completely quietly or doing something where I'm not reporting to someone: not answering the phone, not getting something for someone, just locking myself away. Taking a bubble bath, even a mental bubble bath.

Gary: What's been your best source of reliable information as a caregiver?

Dana: Other caregivers. Over the past few years, I've talked to a lot of women whose husbands are injured, sharing tips and ideas, and venting with one another. You get advice from your doctors, or you get the official recommended procedure on some things, and then someone else will come in and say, "Oh, you know what's easier?" Or they'd say, "Well yes, you can spend all this money on this particular kind of bandage, or you can cut up a Maxi pad and it sticks to the sock." I get all of this useful information about so many different products that are helpful. Everything from machines to suppositories.

Gary: How do you redefine "normality" in your life?

Dana: I think it becomes easier as you become used to it. The first year anniversary was very, very tough because every landmark we hit, I remembered the year before when it wasn't that way.

The second anniversary was easier, because I was looking back on the first year and how tough that was. Then this past year went by, and we've been able to look back and think, "We've come really far. Things are becoming positive and definitely different."

But, there's also some wonderful stuff that comes out of it. I mean meeting people we may never have met, and strangely enough, opportunities that may never have been taken advantage of. Directing is something Chris has always talked about, and then he ended up directing a beautiful film which came directly out of people wanting to reach out and give him opportunities. And he ended up winning awards for it. So, that's something that has come directly out of the tragedy. I'm also grateful for what Chris' injury has done in terms of elevating the consciousness of the country, and the world, about the disabled. He's made a tremendous change in terms of people's awareness.

Gary: You must hear all the time about how heroic you've been. How do you feel about that?

Dana: I'm actually very uncomfortable with that title because I don't feel like a hero. When Chris and I got married, I took my wedding vows very seriously. When I took those vows and said I will be there in sickness and in health, no matter what, that was a scary day. That was the day when I said, "Okay, here we go. We're going on this journey, and let's hope it's a fun one." Really, it has been.

As far as my situation today, I don't see any other choice. I don't say that in a negative way. It's just not a situation where there is a choice. I'm so grateful that I have the stuff to be able to cope with difficult times. I credit my parents for that. But let's be honest, we have financial resources that many, many people don't have. I was very happy living in a kind of obscure existence. Then, suddenly, Chris is in the limelight. The upside of that is I get support in droves, so I don't see myself as particularly heroic.

I do see many, many caregivers, mostly women, every day, who are the real heroes. People who really have a struggle, who are invisible and not in the limelight. Their husbands are irrevocably depressed and have not been able to get back to work. These women are doing what I'm doing, but have a job that is a thousand times harder. If people say I'm a hero, I'm glad they think, "Okay, caregiver equals hero." But personally, I have it much easier than many people, and I certainly do this out of love and commitment. I also recognize that there's a trap in the perception of caregivers: we do these things out of love and, therefore, we have to do it without any rights. I don't think that's fair.

Gary: Chris mentioned in *Still Me* that only 30 percent of people will fight their insurance company. Do you have any advice for the other 70 percent?

Dana: Yes. My first piece of advice is, "Don't take it personally." When I first started fighting the insurance company, I used to scream and cry, "How can they be doing this to us?" Then I realized they do it to everybody. My second piece of advice is, when people ask, "Can I do anything to help?", assign them writing letters to the insurance companies after you get denials. Writing re-submissions becomes an incredibly valuable thing that someone can do for you. It's amazing how much it will ease your mind. Whenever someone asks if they can help me, I ask them to do something specific, and it gets done. I think that people want to help, even busy people.

Gary: Tell me about the Christopher Reeve Foundation?

Dana: The mission of the foundation is two-fold: to support scientific research towards a cure for paralysis, and to give out what we call Quality of Life Grants. These are for people with disabilities in areas of caregiving, transportation, recreation, personal needs—all different things. We can't give to individuals, but we do give to grassroots organizations. Last year, we gave $100,000 in grants to organizations, including the National Family Caregivers Association. We're a tiny foundation, and we don't have a big staff. A lot of our fundraising has been just by people sending in money and earmarking it for the foundation.

GARY'S NOTE: ROBERT URICH

Robert Urich will always have a special place in my heart as the keynote speaker at our first Fearless Caregiver Conference, which was held in 1998, and for the heroic and very public way he discussed his cancer diagnosis and his incredible rendition of the song *Dulcinea* from the play *Man of La Mancha*. His extremely professional voice shocked the audience who were a little concerned when an action star told them he would like to sing, and then effectively left us all in tears.

But the reason I remember him best was his personal kindness at that event. During the press conference, amid the bank of television cameras and print reporters yelling out questions, he spent time making funny faces at my 12-year-old niece who sat across the room from him, shocked by all the commotion. A very nice guy who was well remembered during another Fort Lauderdale Fearless Caregiver Conference four years later, which coincidentally was held on the day he passed away.

INTERVIEW WITH ROBERT URICH

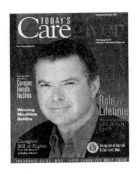

SEPT / OCT 1997

Gary Barg: Most people go through things like cancer privately; you didn't. Did dealing with it in public make a difference for you?

Robert Urich: What I unknowingly did was unleash this army of support. I got letters and telegrams from Jay Leno, Steven Cannell and a few of those kinds of people, and then I got letters and calls from people all over the world. If I had to give anybody a bit of advice, I would say, "Don't go through this alone."

First of all, I was too frightened to go through it alone. I didn't think that was a burden I wanted to carry alone. Joseph Conrad, the writer and poet, said, "We live as we dream, alone." Ultimately when the lights are turned out and it's 2 o'clock in the morning, everybody's asleep in the house and you can hear the little pump from the chemo pumping its magic into your body, it's a lonely, scary time. You do go through that by yourself. But I'm quite confident that sharing this experience with my family and friends, and my extended family, and the fans around the country who wrote—I received over 50,000 pieces of mail—I'm sure that created a surge of positive energy which allowed me to get better, faster. I really think that's why I was able to handle this as well as I did.

Also, I wanted to be a partner with my doctors. I didn't want to be a patient. I didn't want to be a victim or place blame, you know, "Why did this happen to me?" I learned a long time ago, as soon as you place blame, you make yourself a victim and you empower someone else with taking over your life.

So I allowed myself 48 hours of shock and emotions. Friends would call and ask if I was going to the ball game. I would say "No, I can't," and they would ask "Why not?" I'd start to cry, but come Monday morning, that stopped. The doctors said I should start the treatment right away. I asked to have the weekend to collect myself, to mentally plan this. They said I could wait that long. They opened at 6:00 a.m., Monday, and I said "Well, I'll be there at 10 to 6:00 because I want to be the first one to be cured." That's how I went about it, in a very businesslike kind of way.

Gary: How did you approach the fear?

Robert: Head on. I've always played these characters who have been capable and up to the challenge, no matter what it was, and I thought, well, maybe it's time for me to see if I can display some of that toughness. I took it one step at a time. I think I've always had this strong faith and belief in a higher power and you have to surrender to that, too; that's how I did it.

Gary: How did all this affect your children?

Robert: Well, Ryan was out on a National Outdoor Leadership trip for 30 days in the wilderness, so he didn't know what was going on. When he came home, my wife drove to Lander, Wyoming, and waited for the bus to come out of the mountains so that he didn't hear about it from the radio or some newscaster or the cover of some magazine. Emily was at school, and we insisted she finish. When she came home, she came straight to the hospital. When Emily saw me hooked up to all the stuff, she got a little upset. They were both going away to boarding school because that's what they wanted, but now they've decided to come home and finish up in Los Angeles. I have my family back; we're all living under the same roof. I think it caused them both to grow up a little bit and mature a little bit, and face this notion of mortality, which is extremely difficult, I would think, for teenagers to do. But, we're back together, and I know for me, it's been a tremendous source of growth and inspiration. There's a famous quotation by Carl Jung, the Swiss psychologist, who said, "Conflict"—and this indeed has been a source of conflict for my family and me—"engenders fire: the fire of passions and effects. And like all fire, it has two properties, that of combustion and that of creating light." I thought if I could somehow survive the combustion aspect of this event, maybe it could be a source of illumination for me, and growth; and I must say that it has.

Gary: How were you able to help the kids through their fears?

Robert: We didn't keep anything from them. We made sure they knew exactly what was going on at all times. When I was doing the chemo, I started to lose my hair. It was coming out in chunks, and I just did not want to deal with that. So I sent my son to pick up a pair of electric shears, and he shaved all the hair off—what was left. That kind of de-mystified it for him. We laughed about it and joked about how I could do all those Yul Brenner parts. I think constant communication helped us through it.

There was one other thing. While Emily was still at school, Ryan came home early. He drove me to chemo courses and he worked at the cancer center and learned about what was going on. He helped in the office and put stickers on envelopes for them, so he was right there with me while I was going in for my treatments. He was actually doing something. He volunteered and did some community service.

Gary: A lot of people get to the point where they feel like the victim and their whole life just stops. You had those first 48 hours, but then you turned it around. How?

Robert: Well, I think that's the way I've always lived my life. I learned those lessons long ago, in other aspects of my life. You control the stuff you can control. We've all heard that. There's a quote, and it's not original, but Steven Covey says it in his *Seven Habits of Highly Effective People* and Kathleen Brehony in her book, *Awakening at Midlife* (which is a wonderful book I highly recommend), says it—We can't always control our destiny, but we certainly can control how we react to what happens to us. I just know that to be true.

Gary: How has your life changed since you had cancer?

Robert: Well, I think the hardest part right now is to NOT think about it all day long. Psychologically, it left a tremendous scar, and every day I wake up and take an inventory of how I feel and what's going on in my body. Every day, it's "Ohhh…what is that ache and pain? Is that because I played too many holes of golf, or is that something I need to worry about? Prior to this event, I would have aches and pains and not think anything of it. But I have to just move on. So I think, psychologically, the healing takes a little longer than the physical healing.

Gary: Has this experience affected your faith at all?

Robert: I think I'm closer to the Supreme Being in my daily life now than I ever was when I was going to church every Sunday when I was young. My spirituality has matured over a period of years and it's grown. I was not hesitant to think about God and entrusting my life to a higher power.

Gary: Do you do any meditation or use any visualization?

Robert: Absolutely; I firmly believe there is a connection between mind and body. I don't know if I take it so far as some of these guys being able to cause things to happen. I just used a certain kind of visualization as a relaxation exercise for myself. I used it like a golden light Roto-Rooter. I would create this image I have, of a favorite spot of mine where the sun hits the lake late in the afternoon. It just turns golden, and I let that light come into the top of my head and swirl around every inch of my brain and my head, down through my body and into my arms and legs. As this golden light went swirling around, I imagined it destroying whatever bad cells or bad things that were in my body and just go whooshing around at the bottom of my feet and being gone. I actually tried to create positive images of good coming in and bad going out. That made a difference in the way I felt about things. I felt like I was doing something to make myself better and maybe that's the most important thing.

Gary: What would you say is the most important piece of advice you'd like to leave family caregivers?

Robert: I think that what we must remember is that all we have is today—this moment. And love each other, support and take care of each other. It works both ways. I thought, even though I was the sick one, I felt a need to try and be as normal as I could and contribute to the relationship. Don't just sit around and let people wait on you hand and foot. We have to take charge of what's going on in our lives, even when we're not feeling very well.

INTERVIEW WITH ART LINKLETTER

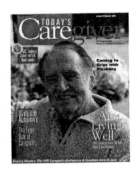

JAN / FEB 1998

Gary Barg: You describe yourself as a messenger of "Positive Aging." What does that mean?

Art Linkletter: That means that in the face of all the negative stereotypes about how anyone over the age of 60 is either sick or senile or sexless, I'm living proof that that's not so. At 85, I travel a couple of hundred thousand miles a year, I speak about 70 times a year, I've got a new series on the air with Bill Cosby starting in January, and during the intervals, I ski and surf. So that proves you don't have to feel that when you reach 60 or above, you are destined to be chronically ill, depressed or useless. I talk about my life and my philosophy to many different kinds of groups.

Gary: Tell me about your seven rules to grow older by.

Art: If you want to live longer and be better, or as I say it, "Be better and live longer," whether you are the caregiver or the person receiving care, above everything else, if you're smoking, stop smoking or using tobacco. You must have moderation in alcohol. You must have a low fat diet with plenty of fiber and fruit to go with it. You must have seven to nine hours of sleep. You must have a good breakfast, and you must exercise at least three or four times a week, for 15 to 20 minutes, moderately. Finally, you must exercise your mind with positive thinking, and by being interested in learning and using your brain.

Gary: Is there any one malady you have seen affect older caregivers the most?

Art: Depression is the old folks' single greatest enemy, outside of chronic health diseases like cancer and heart. There are millions of Americans who feel depression because they are lonely. They feel out of the loop. They are lost. They feel bored, without purpose, and depression sets in. And as it sets in, we now know, it affects the immune system. And that opens the door to a lot of problems you just don't want to have.

Gary: You have visited over 200 nursing homes. What have you learned from those visits which might be useful for caregivers?

Art: I've learned there are as many varieties of nursing homes as there are varieties of barbecued pork ribs. You can have from the barest, skimpiest non-caring giving to the loving, warm, kind caring that is the dream of every person who gets older. Nursing homes have become a terror for many older people. They fear they are going to be neglected by their family, once they are put there, and as they get older. Kind of out of sight, out of mind, but more importantly, that they're going to be neglected by the people who are working there. I would have my relatives, or whoever, drop in at unannounced hours before I ever went there, to see if things were all that they are supposed to be and talk to other people there. Ask them what they thought of the food, and what they thought of the care. If they need something, and they rang the bell, did someone show up, or did they wait a couple of hours? Really, you have to do some research.

Gary: Did you develop a rule of thumb, so that when you walked into a facility you had an idea of what it was going to be like?

Art: First of all, is it clean? Are there any smells or odors, do the people seem happy? There is an aura of happiness that exists in a well-run nursing home. The people living there are smiling, they're laughing, they're happy. And at other places, they are almost comatose. Generally speaking, you want a place where their employees and volunteers are spiritual people. You will find that those people do not have a job when they help you, they have a calling. The people who are working in nursing homes, and especially of all places, hospice, must have belief in God and a belief in the goodness of people to do the right job, because it's so thankless. In many cases, particularly when 30 to 40 percent of the people have dementia of one kind or another, you don't get thanked. You don't even get a smile. They don't even know you the next time they see you. This calls for a special kind of feeling that is often present, although not always, in people who have a deep spiritual conviction.

Gary: What do you say to caregivers when you speak with them?

Art: I've done lectures and seminars for caregivers on the topic of "burnout." Burnout can affect everybody. No matter who you are, you wear out. You wear down, and have to have ways to fight that! You have to take vacations, find ways of creating fun and laughing, of looking for humor. You have to combat burnout the way you would physical exhaustion. There are many ways you can do this. You have to have ways of relieving and releasing pressure and resentment, and the feeling of being overworked and not appreciated. And that's being with other people. Don't be alone; get out for a couple of hours, get away for a day or two, where laughter and fun and life are all around you. Caregivers can and do get together in groups and talk about their problems, so that it isn't all bottled up. Everybody has the right to sit around and complain once in a while about the little old lady in room 24 who spits in your face when you lean over to say hello. And then you can laugh together about it. And now you have something known as the Sandwich Generation, where the kids have come back to live with the parents, and the grandparents are there, too. Caregivers find they have to bend over backwards to acknowledge that the other generation is different: different language, different thoughts, and different values. You can't be whining, carping and moaning, trying to change them. Just be an example. That's the best way. Be serene and happy. Try to be indifferent to things that are difficult. That's what positive thinking is all about. It's not easy with all the negativity around us. But you can't husband your sorrow; you have to let it go.

Gary: What should caregivers know about seniors and sex?

Art: In the first place, people still have every kind of emotion that they've ever had. And they're not to be embarrassed or poked fun at even if they have intimate relations at an advanced age. I also want to point out that sex is a whole lot more than physical. It is intimacy.

It can be flirting, complimenting, doing little things like leaving little notes for someone. Caregivers should encourage this without promoting unreal situations. But mostly, they shouldn't put down or embarrass older people for having these relationships.

INTERVIEW WITH ED MCMAHON

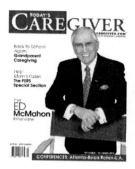

NOV / DEC 2003

Gary Barg: What has been your experience with being a family caregiver?

Ed McMahon: My son Michael became very sick. He was traveling on the East Coast and taking a break between gigs, and he kept complaining to me about his back. I told him that he's got to see a doctor, and he kept saying he would. Finally, when he traveled out West and got to my house, he was green. I took him to my doctor as soon as possible. Sadly, we found out that he had cancer.

Gary: What happened next?

Ed: It was too late at this point. It had started in his colon and had spread throughout his body. I moved him in with us, and all we could do was give him care. The guest bedroom became like a hospital room, with a hospital bed, nurses around the clock, and we gave him the best care that we could. It took about six months for the cancer to kill him. One thing that I was very impressed with was hospice, and how they took over. I have high praise for hospice because they included everyone in the family.

Gary: What should caregivers know about the Muscular Dystrophy Association and what it accomplishes through the telethon?

Ed: It is my 36th year with the Jerry Lewis Telethon, and what it accomplishes is that 90 percent of the money it receives actually goes into care, devices, and research. The money is so well used. The charity gets awards every year for how well the money is used and spent on the actual needs of those who suffer. The researchers are trying to penetrate the medical mystery of where these diseases come from and what causes them. Each year, it's gratifying because our medical men will announce a breakthrough of some kind. There are 40 diseases involved with this, and so there's a lot to cover, and it's great to know that breakthroughs are being made all the time.

Gary: I'm glad that you brought up the 40 other diseases. I know that people always think of just muscular dystrophy, but there are all these other branches to this illness.

Ed: Yes, the most famous of them is Lou Gehrig's disease, but there are 39 other diseases with names that I can't pronounce and they are just as bad.

Gary: I know you are also on the board of the St. Jude's Ranch.

Ed: Yes, it's right outside Las Vegas, in Henderson.

Gary: I'm a big fan of what they do at St. Jude's Hospital, but I wasn't familiar with the ranch.

Ed: They have a similar name, but they are not the same organization. The ranch takes in abused children. St. Jude, being the patron saint of the hopeless, makes a great name for different organizations. St. Jude's in Memphis is a wonderful facility and organization unto its own.

Gary: Any advice that you have for family caregivers?

Ed: There is no training for it. You have to jump into it pretty quickly, and learn by trial and error. You should know where the closest hospice is, just as you know where the nearest hospital is, because there's a fair chance that someone in your family will need to call upon those services in your lifetime; maybe even you.

▪ GARY'S NOTE: DIXIE CARTER

Actress, comedienne, singer, Broadway star and caregiver, Ms. Dixie was best known for her scene stealing role as Julia Sugarbaker on the television program *Designing Women*. Dixie was also a song stylist, critically acclaimed as a cabaret performer. Few people knew that she was also a family caregiver. She cared first for her beloved father Cart and then for her aunt, both in her home in California as well as in her hometown of McLemoresville, Tennessee.

Dixie spoke in a mellifluous and genteel whisper during the entire cover interview with me for *Today's Caregiver* magazine. She possessed the kind of southern gentility where she would refer to her husband as Mr. Hal Holbrook in conversation, as opposed to my husband or simply Hal. That was one conversation that I really didn't want to end. I appreciated her frankness and honesty about her family caregiving; I think she was extremely interested in helping other caregivers through what she had encountered. She was very appreciative of the hospice staff that helped her father in the end and wanted to make sure that caregivers fully understood the value of hospice care. I hope that she didn't think I was disinterested in our conversation since I was sure she could hear snoring on my end of the phone. We had just received a new puppy, who was sleeping in my lap (to keep him quiet). That didn't work so very well since he snored loudly throughout the entire interview.

INTERVIEW WITH DIXIE CARTER

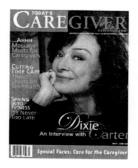

MAY / JUN 2007

Gary Barg: I'm so very sorry to hear about your father's passing. You had been his caregiver for some time before he passed. Was it a difficult transition for him to move out to Los Angeles?

Dixie Carter: Of course it was, but he handled it in the way he handled things, which was he didn't make anyone aware of it. He and my mother were very much a part of raising my children because of my divorce from the father of my children; I called upon them, and on all my family, for various kinds of support and assistance. When I moved out to California, my parents would come out and they would stay on, so the connection there was very strong. My mother died out here in Los Angeles in 1988. The truth was, I didn't think Daddy would live 15 minutes after my mother died. I thought that grief would cut him down, and I feared for him. That was the reason why I wanted him to live with me. I dreaded it because I thought that I would not have my own grief over my mother, but I felt like that's what needed to happen to give him any kind of a chance for a life after he lost her. My children actually got down on their knees, bent down by his chair, and said, "Cart"—all his grandchildren called him Cart for Albert Carter—they said, "Cart, Momma needs you. You have to go live with her now." It was so sweet, so moving. So, he agreed to come live with me, but I really didn't become a caregiver for a long time. He lived with me for 15 years before care was needed.

Gary: When did you actively start to care for him?

Dixie: My father's father had had Parkinson's disease, and so we both knew something was coming on. It started to affect the way that he walked, and it was very difficult to get him to actually exercise. The trembling was getting worse. He'd have to have a certain amount of physical therapy. He would walk, and he would really make the effort to do so, but it was becoming more and more difficult. I want to say this to all of your readers: being in a house with family is home, wherever it is; being in a house with someone you love, someone who loves you enough that they want to share the same domicile with you is in itself a social connection. It's company; it's its own kind of comfort and not exactly a lonely existence. You could be in a facility with other people your age, but still be very lonely; but being in the home with one of your children, one of your own, is comforting and so loving, that the attention that I had believed I would need to give, by sitting down and conversing on a daily basis for some length, turned out not to be necessary.

Gary: That's so very important. I always say that caregiving is such a family issue, and on the flipside of that, kids seeing their parents caring for a loved one is a life lesson that they will pass down to the next generation.

Dixie: I'm not saying that it's easy. When someone goes into the stage where they need physical care, it can be very hard. When I was in New York two years ago, I was on the phone with my father who was in Los Angeles, and he said to me, "Precious, I think I'm starting to get some dying illness. I think it's time for me to go back to Tennessee." I said, "Yes, Sir, as soon as we leave New York." My husband,

Hal Holbrook, and I moved lock, stock and barrel back with my father to his home. Not many people have that extraordinary luxury or gift, to have the home they were born in to be still standing. He went back there and was not able to walk by the time we arrived. Then these angels came into our lives; angels who were in and around the area, who came in and took eight hour shifts. This one man who worked for me, Juan Castillo, was tremendously attached to my father and volunteered to move in with him. Along with the young man who tended to the garden and the grounds, together they would lift my father into his wheelchair so he could go in and get his breakfast. This all happened out of love and by people whose job wasn't to do this kind of work, and I couldn't have done it without them.

Gary: Was hospice involved in the last days?

Dixie: Hospice came in during the last couple of weeks. There was never any emphasis on, "How long is this going to take?" or "We can't be doing this forever." I thought when hospice came in, a doctor had to declare that the patient was terminally ill.

Gary: The wonderful thing about hospice care is that they are there as long as the process goes on.

Dixie: I have to say that in addition to this extraordinary love that my father received from his caregivers in Tennessee, they also turned out to be wonderfully careful. When my father passed away, and he'd been pretty much in that bed for two and a half years, he did not have a single bed sore, and that only comes from an extraordinary love of what you are doing. Hospice came in, and I experienced the same thing, the same quality, and the same feelings from them. I think that, in general, people aren't aware that this is available to them.

Gary: When people like you talk about their experience with hospice, it helps overcome the misinformation and the lack of knowledge about the process. You've done a lot to help really busy people learn about yoga and healthy living, and I guess there is no one busier than a family caregiver. What can you share with caregivers about taking care of themselves?

Dixie: When my father died, also living in the house was my mother's baby sister Helen, who had a stroke last August. She's now here in Los Angeles. She got here a week ago, and she was accompanied by one of the ladies from hospice who had been looking after my father and her. She's in my father's old room, and it's the only way I could think of that she could be well taken care of. It's been a very emotional thing for me. It just seems like sometimes it's just more than enough. I don't do the hands-on caring, but I am very present. I stay on top of the medications, and I pick out what she would wear today, and make sure that things are going alright. So, the folks who work for me here have taken on this additional job and I have discovered that my back is in knots—completely in knots! Since I made this decision, my back has been totally out. I just started realizing over the past couple of days that if I want these muscle spasms to stop, I'm going to have to back emotionally away from this a little bit, and go out and find some breathing time. I go to church and I depend on prayer a lot. I think that there is a need to get more rest than what would usually serve you.

Gary: I think that is such an important point, and frankly, hands-on or not, you are a family caregiver and you have all the stress.

Dixie: I have all of the responsibility and it's very weighty. I'm realizing that with my father's death, the tremendous weakness that comes with grief has not prepared me for having to make this decision about the one remaining person from that generation that I'm still close to. So, hospice has come out here, and they really have stepped in; they've been here from the get-go. Yesterday, a social worker from hospice was here, and the day before that, the chaplain was here. There are all kinds of wonderful helpers who come from hospice. The day after my aunt got here, the wind was blowing so hard where we live that the lights went out for 24 hours and it was not pleasant. I cleverly lit a bunch of candles and got the fires going in the fireplaces because without the power, we had no heat and Helen seemed to have a bad reaction to the morphine that had been prescribed for her. She was weakening and her heart was beating badly, and I thought that maybe we should give her some oxygen; but then I looked around at all the candles and fires going and I said that she was just going to have to make it without some. We managed to place a chair in a hallway, away from everything, and gave some oxygen. So we've had our times, and through this all-night vigil, hospice was right here and never deserted us.

Gary: That's great that you knew to call them and get them involved during all of that.

Dixie: It creates an absolute bond and a deep understanding—the "words that lie too deep for tears." If you go through and experience life and death together, you are united, in a mystical and highly spiritual way. The person who is being cared for is in trouble; he or she knows that they're in trouble, there's no getting around it; otherwise, none of this would be going on. It's a very hard time, and the shared experience helps people not to feel so lonely. Sometimes I felt so alone in just trying to hold down the fort, because I saw that my father's health was deteriorating and I was so lonely and frightened. When I got to Tennessee and saw that he had caregivers there, the sense of absolute aloneness changed in me.

Gary: What would you say is the most important piece of advice you'd like to leave family caregivers?

Dixie: Caregiving will be unlike anything you will do in your whole life; it's a different endeavor from any other endeavor in life. You, the person doing it, get something very rich; a great, great learning experience. My advice would be to try; say your prayers and try, and believe that there will be a response to your needs. Believe that as unlikely as it may seem to you, there will be a response to your needs; don't be afraid to ask for it. Try.

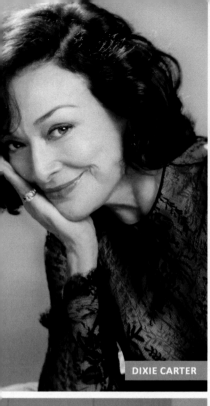

DIXIE CARTER

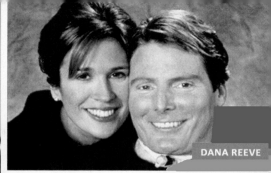

DANA REEVE

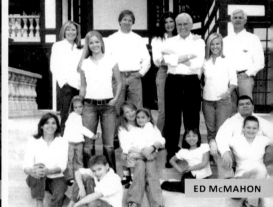

ED McMAHON

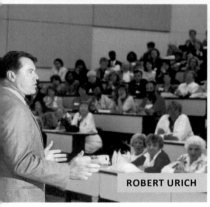

ROBERT URICH

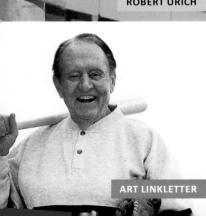

ART LINKLETTER

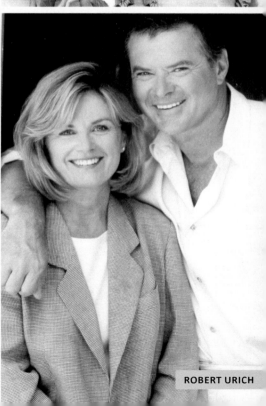

ROBERT URICH

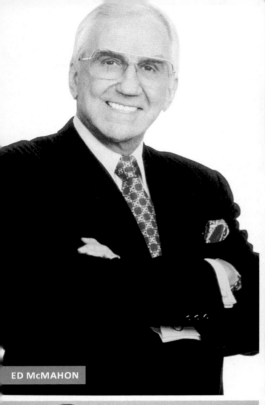

ED McMAHON

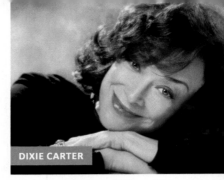

DIXIE CARTER

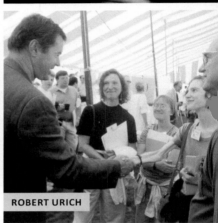

ROBERT URICH

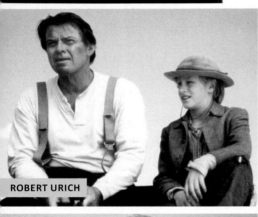

ROBERT URICH

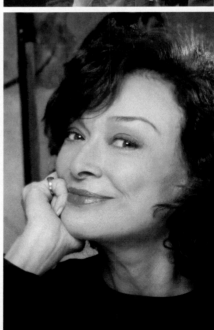

DIXIE CARTER

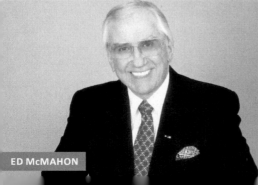

ED McMAHON

ABOUT THE AUTHOR

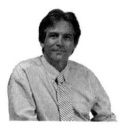

A noted speaker, writer and publisher on caregiving issues since 1995, Gary Barg is founder and editor-in-chief of *Today's Caregiver* magazine and caregiver.com.

Gary also created The Fearless Caregiver Conferences, hosted across the country, which bring together family and professional caregivers to share their knowledge and experience. His first book, *The Fearless Caregiver,* is filled with practical advice, caregiver poetry and inspirational stories. Since 2001, *Today's Caregiver* magazine has conducted the annual Caregiver Friendly Awards highlighting the year's best products and services designed to enhance the lives of family caregivers.

Gary started his career as a caregiver advocate in 1994 while visiting his mother, who was caring for his grandparents in Miami. While there, he became concerned for his mother's own health and well-being. He relocated to South Florida and became a caregiver's caregiver, caring for her as she cared for her parents. After months of seeking information they needed as family caregivers, he created *Today's Caregiver* magazine and caregiver.com, both launched in 1995. He remains on the road throughout the year, talking with caregivers at Fearless Caregiver Conferences and as a keynote speaker at many other events, helping caregivers learn all they can about their role as CEO of Caring for Their Loved One, Inc.